THE COOR OF LIGHT

DAILY MEDITATIONS FOR ALL OF US
LIVING WITH AIDS

THE COLOR OF LIGHT

DAILY MEDITATIONS FOR ALL OF US LIVING WITH AIDS

PERRY TILLERAAS

Illustrations by
David Spohn

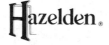

First published October, 1988.

ISBN: 0-89486-511-0

Printed in the United States of America
Library of Congress Catalog Card Number 88-81907

Editor's Note:
  Hazelden Educational Materials offers a variety of information on chemical dependency and related areas. Our publications do not necessarily represent Hazelden or its programs, nor do they officially speak for any Twelve Step organization.

ACKNOWLEDGMENTS

Because this book comes from a collective experience, it is impossible to thank everyone responsible. However, credit for the fact that it exists at all is due to the wonderful people at Hazelden Educational Materials. I am grateful for their interest and for their faith in me. Thanks especially to my editor, Becky Post, for her constant support.

Thanks to all the people who allowed me to quote them and to everyone who shared their experience, strength, and hope with me. Thanks to my friends in PWAlive, to Morgan for being a constant cheerleader, to my parents who are proud of me, and to all those people who, one day at a time, help me stay clean and sober. Thanks to my spirit guides who hover near my right shoulder and are responsible for much of what, in these pages, is inspired or helpful.

Thank you to Walter, who long ago told me about a strange disease that was killing his friends. Often, while writing this book, I have felt your presence. I still miss you.

Finally, thank you to all people with AIDS. You are teachers for our planet. This book is dedicated to you.

INTRODUCTION

There is an old native North American Indian tradition called Heyoehkah. The Heyoehkahs, or sacred clowns, were people within the tribe who "did things differently," challenged people's thinking, shook them up. Their function was to keep their people from getting stuck in rigid ways of thinking and living. They were also known as "contraries" because they lived backwards. They walked backward, danced backward, everything they did was contrary to the norm. By their living, they symbolized the shadow of the Creator God, reminding people of their spiritual center.

For gay people, the role of Heyoehkah is especially important: not only are Heyoehkahs often gay, the role of contrary is a sacred symbol of the role we play among society as a whole.

Not long ago, a handsome, courageous, young, gay Indian named Richard, danced Heyoehkah at a powwow. When I heard about it, shivers ran down my spine. It was a sign of remembering. It was a sign that we are remembering our relation to the Great Spirit and that the Creator God is remembering us.

His dance also made me realize that from the beginning there has been a Heyoehkah response to AIDS. When the normal response was to react with fear and panic, there were people dancing backward, responding with love and confidence.

When, every day, the world began repeating a death mantra, our sacred clowns danced the dance of life. They talked about living with AIDS, surviving, healing, recovering. When the normal reaction to a diagnosis was isolation, our Heyoehkahs dragged us into a community. When the world wanted us to be victims, they drew circles of light around themselves and stood in their power.

Whenever it got dark, they turned toward the light. Whenever people said there is no hope, they said there is always hope. Whenever people said this isn't about us, they stood up and said, "This *is* about you. This is about us all. Our planet is sick. Earth has acquired an immune dysfunction. We are all living with AIDS."

The heart of this book is inspired by that magical AIDS community of sacred clowns, the contrary people who keep hope alive, who stay spirit-centered, who "do things differently."

PERRY TILLERAAS

January

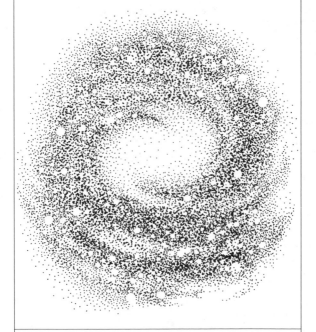

I am connected to the one source of all light. So are my friends. I feel their peaceful presence and trust they feel mine.

We give thanks for unknown blessings already on their way.
— *Sacred Ritual Chant*

Too often we think we have to earn the blessings of the universe. We think if we do enough of the right things, we will be protected, maybe even rewarded. The problem is, we never know what's enough so we always try to do a little more. It's a very adult way of viewing the world but not much fun.

Young children have a better way of looking at life. They expect wonderful gifts just because they're children, not because they are "naughty or nice."

We have a choice. We can be worrisome adults or children of the universe.

Wonderful gifts are coming my way today. I don't have to do anything to deserve them. They are coming to me just because I live. I expect them and am open to receiving them. I wonder what magic the world has in store for me today.

The clue is not to ask in a miserly way
— the key is to ask in a grand manner.
— Ann Wigmore

How expansive can we be today? How grand? Can we ask for the sun, moon, and stars? Can we ask for what we really, really, in our heart of hearts, want?

"What do I want?" This is probably the hardest question we can ask ourselves. And it's an important question to answer because it determines how we live our lives. Think about it for a while. It's an important enough question to spend the entire day thinking about, dreaming about, reaching deep inside, and discovering what we really want.

Once we know what we want, we can boldly affirm ourselves and our right to be everything we can be, to be our true creative, divine selves. We can open our chests, throw our shoulders back and say out loud, this is what I want.

The world is abundant and the more we have, the more we have to share. The more light in our lives, the more light in the world.

Today I will decide what I really want, and I will ask for it. I will be expansive and generous to myself.

The life of man is divided between waking, dreaming, and dreamless sleep. But transcending these three states is superconscious vision — called the Fourth.
— from the Upanishads

Many of us have had spiritual or mystical experiences that we are hesitant to share with others. Our fear of being made fun of keeps us isolated in that very important area of our lives. But when we do share some of our deepest feelings about "what it all means" we are often happily surprised to discover that our friends have had similar experiences.

When we deny our spiritual selves we get out of balance. To heal we must recover our balance and pay attention to all areas of our lives — physical, mental, emotional, and the Fourth, spiritual.

Each of us gets to discover our own spirituality. We needn't be bound to the religion of our childhoods. In the end, we are totally free to find our own path. We are responsible only to our own intuition, to our higher self.

I honor the spiritual beliefs of my brothers and sisters and in return am supported and respected for who I am and what I believe.

We didn't just begin to love when AIDS came along. We have been loving for a very long time.

— Kal

AIDS brings many of us together in loving unity. It challenges us to love each other unconditionally. Because of AIDS, we are learning to see beyond the surface and getting to know the real person. We are developing loving support systems. We have real friends, not just drinking buddies.

And yet, it is important to remember that all of us have been loving for a very long time. We've been demonstrating courage, compassion, and care for a long time too. We didn't just start with AIDS.

We've been parents, teachers and nurses, social workers, and caregivers. We've been uncles and brothers, sisters and daughters. We've been poets, actors, doctors, and healers. We've been singing and dancing and loving as hard as we could. And we've had the courage to openly love each other in the face of bigotry and hatred.

Now AIDS gives us a chance to teach the world what we've learned about love, hope, courage, and compassion.

I cherish all my experiences. They bring me to where I am today. I am grateful for being who I am.

*The immune system is affected positively
and negatively by thoughts and feelings.*
— Mark Friedlander and Terry Phillips

Stress, fear, tension, and anxiety keep our bodies
busy producing all kinds of hormones. When we
are stressed out, all our endocrine glands go to work
except our thymus gland, home base for our immune system and major T cell producer. It shuts
down. In fact, our entire immune system shuts
down when we're upset. Worry, anger, dread, resentment, all contribute to a weaker defense system.

The good news is that a bright attitude, thoughts
of love, security, safety, healing, sunshine, and
feelings of joy and relaxation all contribute to a
strengthened immune system. We have the power
to choose which thoughts to hang on to and which
thoughts to let go. When negative thoughts appear,
we can let them pass like clouds across the sky
and replace them with positive images that make
us smile.

---

*My mind and my body are beautifully connected. I
choose thoughts and experience feelings that strengthen
my wonderful immune system. I love my body. I love
my mind.*

The only way to heal is to be healed.
— *A Course in Miracles*

There are not two classes of people: patients and healers. We are all patients and healers. And all we really have to share is our experience, strength, and hope. Many of us who are chemically dependent and have found relief in a Twelve Step program know how important it is to help others and "carry the message." It is important for them and for us.

But we also know that we can only help someone journey down the road as far as we've gone ourselves. So the most important thing we can do to help others heal is to keep on healing ourselves.

When our focus is always on someone else, the group, or the crisis, and we forget our healing, our program, we are unable to help very much. Now, AIDS is our great teacher. Whether we have a diagnosis or not, we all must find the place where AIDS lives in our lives and begin to heal ourselves there. The more healing we accept for ourselves, the more healing there is in the world.

I accept healing for myself. I allow myself to be healed.

*. . . man can only become what he is able
consciously to imagine, or more precisely,
to "image forth."*

— Dane Rudhyar

All of us have the ability to be wonderfully creative imaginers. And we can use our imaginations to become the people we want to be. The first step is to create a picture in our minds. The next step is to feel it, to imagine the feeling associated with the image.

We can take advantage of the many talented people willing to teach us creative visualization techniques. They can help us develop our ability to visualize and guide us on meditations that can help calm and balance us.

All of us have the ability to visualize. And the more energy we put into positive images, the faster we become powerful self-healers.

We can also "image forth" the world. Imagining ourselves living in a world of peace and love is an important step in making it so.

Today I will use my imagination as a powerful healing tool — for myself and for the entire planet.

*Acting on your love for yourself will include
pursuing people who inspire and excite you.
Assume that you are at least as thrilling
as they are.*
— Christopher Spence and Nancy Kline

Each of us knows people who inspire and excite us. Too often we never approach them because we feel unworthy and are afraid of being rejected. As long as we don't contact them, they won't reject us, but we stay stuck.

Whether our attraction is romantic, intellectual, professional, emotional, or just plain friendly, we demonstrate self-love through action. And approaching people we believe are exciting and thrilling is a great way to prove our love for ourselves.

It doesn't matter what the results are, just as long as we act. Each of us is interesting, thrilling, and exciting. In fact, we're probably attracted to qualities we see in other people that we haven't yet recognized in ourselves.

Today I will make a list of people I want to get to know. I will make at least one phone call. I am not attached to the result. I know that the action itself is life affirming.

*As the soft yield of water cleaves obstinate
  stone,
So to yield with life solves the insoluable:
To yield I have learned is to come back
  again.*

— *Lao Tsu*

Water is a symbol for the feminine side of ourselves. Though society usually associates feminine
with weak and masculine with strong, the reality
is the female part of ourselves makes us very
powerful. Like the moon that controls the oceans,
like water that wears away mountains, the yield-
ing, flowing, intuitive self that we all possess gives
us great strength.

In the past, we thought we had to do it all alone
and that to yield was to give up. Now, in partnership
with others, we know we don't have to do it all
alone. We don't have to have all the answers, and
we don't have to fight all our battles today. Instead,
we have the option to relax and let go. We can let
our Higher Power take over. As we do, the block-
ages, the difficulties, the barriers, and the battles
disappear, dissolve, or become more manageable.

---

*I pray for constant contact with my water self, my
intuitive feminine self, my inner knowingness — my
guide and my strength.*

Accepting the possibility of death —
honestly and completely — frees up a whole
lot of energy to live.
    — Keith Gann, person with AIDS

Until we face the possibility of our death, fear
of dying holds us in its grip. Denial of our fear gives
it tremendous power. It causes us to make decisions based on fear. We glance over our shoulders,
worrying that death is gaining on us. So we run
faster, act more, do more, fret more.

The lessons we learned from facing our addictions can help us face death. We learned that,
though powerless over our addictions, we weren't
helpless. We could call on powerful support from
our friends and from a Higher Power.

AIDS has forced many of us to face our fear of
death. And again we learn that our fears are like
shadows. They disappear in the light. We used to
spend a lot of energy running away from our fears.
Now we can use all that energy to live our lives
wholly and completely in the present.

Today, I will face my fear of death. I will feel the
feelings and experience the pain knowing that I am
totally supported.

*And you who seek to know Me, know that
your seeking and yearning will avail you
not, unless you know the mystery: for if that
which you seek, you find not first within
yourself, you will never find it without.*
— *The Star Goddess from the
Spiral Dance by Starhawk*

Many of us have spent years looking for happiness in the perfect lover, apartment, job, spiritual teacher, sexual experience. We've looked for the secret in books. We thought the right combination of other people's ideas would help us manage our lives. We were always searching, always on the lookout, like someone cruising in a bar. And always we ended up more lonely than before.

The truth is, we already possess everything we need. We carry around our source of wholeness wherever we go. Only when we stop the frantic search for something out there do we realize that the path to happiness leads inside. Only when we slow down and take time to breathe and bring our attention back to our inner selves do we find the love we've been looking for.

I have everything I need. I am filled with abundant energy. I am at peace.

You must feel something to know what it is....

— *Ceanne DeRohan*

Intellectually, we know a lot about AIDS; we know about viruses, T-Cells, vitamins, herbs. But, too often, we don't know how we feel. Many of us have stopped feeling. Long ago, we decided that it was safer not to express our feelings, better to stuff them, better yet to deny having them. We lost our natural talent for feeling and expressing a rainbow of emotions.

Now we can recover our lost feelings. Now we can create a safe space to be totally human. Now our mind and our gut can work together. But they need to learn to like and respect each other first. That's where our heart comes in. Intellect and feeling can join in the heart. The heart is loving; it won't criticize the mind for judging against feeling. It won't criticize feelings for being resentful and afraid of the mind.

I open my heart and allow lost feelings in. My mind is respectful of my feelings. My feelings love my mind. I am grateful for every lost feeling that I can recover.

We all come from the Goddess
And to Her we shall return
Like a drop of rain
Flowing to the ocean.
                    — Sacred Ritual Chant

Every day, many times a day, we come into being and go out of being. We inhale and become filled with breath, life, spirit. We exhale and become empty; life leaves us. The drama of birth and death repeats itself each moment.

We draw breath and are aware of our place in the universe, of our uniqueness, of who we are, and of what our roles are. We let go of breath and are aware of emptiness, nothingness. We are part of the universe then, like a rock, or tree.

We draw breath and are filled with life; we are one with life. We exhale and are separate from all living things. Being, not being. Aware, unaware. United, separate. Inhale, exhale. Birth, death. Transformation.

We are part of a great mystery.

I am one with the earth and all things. I easily and effortlessly come into being and go out of being.

The Will cannot be pressured to forgive before it is really ready because the forgiveness would not be real, but intent to reach forgiveness can allow intense old emotions to move without continuing old hostilities.
— *Original Cause*

We hear a lot about how important forgiveness is to spiritual growth and healing. But old emotions don't go away on their own. They get lodged in our bodies and need to be released. Having intent to forgive brings us to a safe place where we can dislodge resentment and not hurt people.

Intent to reach forgiveness gives us time. It lets us enter a process of releasing rage or hurt or grief and becoming more and more forgiving. Intent to reach forgiveness helps us honestly deal with emotions. We don't have to deny anger just because we think we should be further along spiritually.

Intent to forgive is self-acceptance. It means we stop judging ourselves. It means releasing more and more old emotions, opening more space in our hearts. Space that can then be filled with light and love and true forgiveness.

I accept myself just the way I am. I allow all old emotions to surface. I have intent to forgive. I have intent to heal.

I knew early on I wasn't what they expected. Especially when I got near the age of competitive sports. Then I knew something was way wrong. That's when I really began to take a beating.
— David Grundy

Those of us who are gay took a particularly brutal kind of abuse growing up. After all, the absolutely worst thing anyone could possibly be called was a queer or a faggot.

But all of us, gay or straight, black or white, male or female, can remember feeling different and left out. For many of us it was only when drunk or drugged that we felt like we fit in.

What a joy now to feel unconditional acceptance for being exactly who we are. And what a relief to know that the little boy or girl who felt so alone and was so hurt somehow survived. That little child desperately needs our gentle love and attention. Not one more shaming word. Not one more look of disgust. Only total unconditional love and support. Now we can parent ourselves and make sure we get all the positive attention we need.

Today I will give the little child inside me my total undivided attention and loving support.

*I realize that this diagnosis of AIDS
presents me with a choice: the choice either
to be a hopeless victim and die of AIDS,
or to make my life right now what it always
ought to have been.*
    — *Graham, person with AIDS*

What an incredible challenge — to make our lives
exactly the way we want them to be. The time to
meet this challenge is now. Today. This moment.

What do I want my life to be? How do I express
my true nature, my most creative honest self? How
do I live according to my true purpose? The answers
are usually found in our most secret dreams. Like
frightened animals, they need gentle coaxing to reappear. They need to be reassured that we won't
discount or criticize them.

If our lives don't match our dreams, we need to
act. We need to act in our health care decisions,
in our relationships, in our jobs. AIDS gives us the
opportunity to dramatically change our lives. AIDS
gives us permission to act on our dreams and
desires and become the people we want to be. Now.

---

*Today I will sit quietly and ask my secret dreams and
desires to come to me. I will imagine a picture of my
true self. I will take steps toward making my life the
way I want it to be.*

If one asks for success and prepares for failure, he will get the situation he has prepared for.
— *Florence Scovel Shinn*

"Act as if . . ." When we're trying to make big changes and our faith is low, we're told to act as if we already are the kind of people we want to be.

If we ask for and affirm more happiness in our lives but talk and act like we are undeserving, the universe will pay more attention to our actions. When we ask for health but prepare for sickness, health has a hard time getting through.

When the space between our asking and our expectations gets filled with doubt and fear, we can bring our doubts and fears into awareness, bless them, and gently let them go. Then we can act in a way that affirms abundance in our lives.

We need to surround ourselves with positive people who are also expecting and preparing for good things for themselves and for us. It's important to make sure our friends are on a similar path.

I am preparing for success that is already mine. I give thanks for blessings already on their way.

I'm living with AIDS, not dying of AIDS.
— *Bobbie, person with AIDS*

Sometimes the world seems intent on making an AIDS diagnosis or even contact with an AIDS-associated virus a death sentence. But no matter what the world thinks, we can choose our own point of view. We can focus on dying, or we can put our energy into living.

We choose to be conscious of our connection this moment to the loving energy of the universe that surrounds and empowers us. Every time we inhale, we call on the healing power of that energy to cleanse and vitalize each cell of our bodies. Every time we exhale, we gently, lovingly release all pain, all discomfort, all disease, all foreign bodies.

We know that we are not separate, isolated, helpless victims. We are instead filled with power and we choose to live today, aware that we are important in this world. As we express our true selves, the world is healed and so are we. Every breath can be empowering and used to heal and vitalize our bodies. AIDS is teaching us how to live.

I breathe deeply, and the spirit of the universe fills my heart. I am vibrantly alive.

Thus we find the instrument [for the knowledge of God] in ourselves but we find God everywhere.

— *Rudolph Steiner*

The instrument is prayer and meditation. We don't need to be religious to pray or meditate. In fact, for many of us, religion got in the way of our prayer and meditation.

Now, as we reclaim our spirituality, we can develop a form of prayer and meditation that suits us. We can become more familiar with our Higher Power, or however we understand God. We can become more familiar with ourselves. Through prayer and meditation our hearts grow bigger, our lives richer.

In prayer or meditation, we turn our attention inward so that we are more able to see God all around us. When we become conscious of the presence of spirit in our lives, we become more aware of the presence of spirit in everything around us. Life becomes easier. Our path becomes clearer, and we have the power to reach our goals.

Today I will open my heart in prayer and meditation. All through this day I will be aware of universal light and love in everything I see.

Relinquishing control is the ultimate challenge of the Spiritual Warrior.
— The Book of Runes

Sometimes we're called to leap empty-handed into the void, take a huge risk and let go of parts of ourselves that we are attached to — our egos, our character defects, our old behaviors, our fears.

First, we need to know what holds us back. What do we do and what do we believe that keeps us from growing and becoming our true selves?

Then we need willingness to change, willingness to let go of old ideas, habits, patterns — totally. And finally, we need to ask our Higher Power to remove everything that holds us back. Everything.

We may worry, "But who will I be? Will anyone recognize me? What will happen to my personality? No, I can't do that. I must stay in charge of my world. I'll hang on tighter. My life may not be pretty now, but at least it's familiar."

But, out of resistance comes willingness. Out of fear comes faith. And suddenly we are able to leap, to surrender, to let go.

Today I pray for courage to let go. Take away all those things that stand in my way.

You don't have to get sick to get well.
— Louie Nassaney, person with AIDS

For many of us, our experience with AIDS has given us our first taste of unconditional love. All of a sudden we're surrounded by people who care about us. We live in a loving community. There is something special and extraordinary about being with people with AIDS.

At first, those of us without an AIDS or ARC diagnosis felt uncomfortable. We felt we didn't belong and didn't deserve all that love. Now we know that we don't need a diagnosis to belong and we don't have to be a person with AIDS to reach out and ask for what we need. Being sick isn't a condition for receiving love. Love is ours by divine right. Vibrant health is ours by divine right. So are positive support, encouragement, acknowledgment, and constant affirmation.

And we all deserve lots of hugs and physical attention.

All that is mine by divine right now comes to me in perfectly harmonious ways. I move from health to more glorious health. I am at peace.

This is not a dress rehearsal. This is it.
    — *Tom Cunningham*

Many of us know how to live for tomorrow. It's a theory of life based on fear. We're afraid of the future, so we don't dare live with joy and exuberance today. Today is for making sure tomorrow will be safe. Our lives never really start; the curtain never rises. The best we can hope for is a good dress rehearsal.

But AIDS is here now. How we protect and care for ourselves matters now. Our attitudes and behaviors matter now. We are here now — alive and present. Not only is this moment real, but we're real. Many of us have been lost in booze, other drugs, compulsive sex, or other people's lives for so long that we all but disappeared. It's time to come back.

AIDS brings us back. Sobriety brings us back. And now it's time to live. It's time to be who we always wanted to be and to live the way we really want to live. Today.

I am totally alive and present. Today I will make my life exactly the way I want it to be. I am happy, whole, and complete.

*I come from a place of a lot of self-hate
and self-abuse — alcohol and drugs and
you name it. What a joy now not to be
judging myself for my symptoms.*
        — Anita, person with AIDS

We are all doing the best we can. So it's important not to judge against ourselves when, even with
all our affirmations and health work and spiritual
progress, we get sick or slip back into our old ways
of acting and thinking.

Many of us, when we were using alcohol and
other drugs, were cruel to ourselves, especially after
a drunk, blackout, hangover, or yet another anonymous sexual encounter. Now, we can learn how to
be accepting and loving. The first step is to slow
down and be with ourselves, and be with our feelings. We need to be accepting, forgiving, calm, still,
and present.

From that place of quiet we can listen to what
our bodies are saying. What are these symptoms
about? How can I heal? What can I learn?

What a joy now to be gentle with ourselves. How
wonderful to be in partnership with our bodies in
the healing process.

---

*I totally accept myself. I bless my symptoms as mes-
sengers and teachers. I love myself just the way I am.*

I'm not interested in compassion that is focused on my death. Real compassion supports my living and supports me when I express my true gay self.
— *Peter, person with ARC*

Across the country, churches and other organizations are demonstrating their concern for people with AIDS/ARC by trying to be loving and compassionate. But it isn't always easy to distinguish between energy that supports our living and energy that supports our dying. Much of the compassion around AIDS is really support for our dying.

We need support for living. We need to ask for and demand support for being powerful, rooted, honest, and true to ourselves. We need to support each other when we speak our minds and risk offending our "friends." AIDS challenges us to reach across group boundaries, to listen to others and hear differences and similarities. It challenges us to show respect for each other, to honor each others' ways of expression and being in the world.

I surround myself and my friends in protective white light that deflects all negative and unfriendly energy. I am always in divine safety.

Sitting quietly, doing nothing,
Spring comes, and the grass grows by itself.
  — The Gospel According to Zen

How easy to get caught up in activity. Even the activity of recovery and healing. Those of us not "working" but devoting full time to our health can easily get stressed out by the busyness of being a person with AIDS or ARC.

But each day, in fact many times each day, we can sit quietly and just be. We won't call it meditation because it doesn't need a structure or form, and if we call it meditation we will probably take ourselves too seriously. We'll call it loafing or hanging out. We'll sit or lie in the grass and listen, notice, observe. We'll watch our thoughts pass before us like the clouds.

And we'll remember that we are not alone, we are not the only ones involved in our healing and recovery. We are part of the universe, and the universe cares about us and is willing to help.

Today I will sit quietly and let my body heal. I will do my part and I will give God time to do God's part.

Those who have died have never, never left.
The dead are not under the earth.
They are in the rustling trees.
They are in the groaning woods.
They are in the crying grass.
They are in the mouning rocks.
The dead are not under the earth.
                                        — *Birago Diop*

Like the elderly, we scan the obituaries looking for notices of people we didn't know were sick. Many of the announcements hide AIDS as the cause of death in euphemisms and partial truths — cancer or pneumonia at age 42. The survivor's list often fails to name the lover.

Some of us have been to more funerals than our grandparents. We share an unexplainable sorrow, an emptiness for our collective loss. If we allow it, we can tap the river of tears that flows through our subconscious and empties into our heart. Tears for the people we miss. Tears for all people who suffer. Tears for our planet.

Today I will take time for my tears. Today I will remember the dead and listen for their voices.

*I'm grateful to be part of the experience
of AIDS. Grateful to be connected to so
many people with AIDS. You fill me with
your spirit.*

— Michael

Those of us who have felt our eyes well up with
tears of joy and gratitude while listening to the story
of another person's recovery from drinking and
drugging, recognize the same feelings when we
spend time with people with AIDS or ARC.

Alcohol and other drugs brought many of us to
our knees in complete surrender. In our weakness,
in our admission of powerlessness, we were given
the gift of sobriety and the strength to do the
impossible. In our emptiness and surrender we
were filled with power. And a miracle happened.

Now AIDS, another powerful disease, is bringing
us out of isolation into community, out of hurting
into healing, out of disconnection into connection
with the power of the spirit, out of despair into faith
and belief again in miracles.

_____

*Today I am filled with gratitude. I open my heart and
allow it to be filled with love.*

Life and death
should not be considered as opposites.
It is closer to the truth
to speak of dying as an entrance
rather than an exit.

— *Emmanuel*

Each year, those of us who live in northern climates witness dramatic displays of death and transformation. Leaves fall, the earth turns brown, days shorten, and darkness reigns.

During winter, we live on hope. We believe that spring will come, that crocuses will poke through the snow, days will lengthen, and buds will burst from barren branches and the world will be green again.

Nature tells us there is no beginning, no ending, only a continuum, a cycle. Energy moves, changes, transforms. Our dying will only look like dying to those who haven't died, like winter looks to us in January. Our life energy does not collapse; it changes form as we enter another world of adventure, as we make an entrance again.

I pray that I will be clearheaded, totally present and conscious when I make my entrance again. I don't want to miss a thing.

It's our bodies that do the healing. It's time we own our bodies; illness is not the property of doctors, but belongs to us and plays an important role in our lives.
— *Margo Adair*

We know that doctors don't heal broken bones. They set them in place to be healed. Then, miraculously, our bodies go to work and the bone becomes one again.

In the meantime, we're forced to slow down. We know intuitively that the broken bone is a message. AIDS can be a message too, a big message. Our bodies are trying to get our attention, so we listen as closely as we can and make the changes as best we can.

In other words, we set ourselves in readiness. With the help of our healers, we place ourselves in the best position for our body to heal itself. And if we can, we give thanks for the teaching, for the lesson, for the learning. We honor and respect our body's miraculous ability to heal itself.

I listen to my body. I hear its subtle messages. I thank my illness and let it go. I set my whole self – body, mind, and spirit — in a place that allows me to heal.

*I am a Divine, magnificent expression of
life. I rejoice in my sexuality and in all that
I am. I love myself.*

— *Louise Hay*

I affirm again and again my own divine nature.
Each vision of who I really am powerfully propels
me into becoming all I can be. Each good thing I
do for myself heals the wounds inflicted by my past
self-abusive behavior.

Each kind act heals me. Each time I eat right, each
time I meditate, look in the mirror and smile, call
a friend, or take a walk teaches the little child within
me that I love him or her.

I affirm myself as a sexual being too. I affirm and
acknowledge the wonder that is my body. I honor
my sexuality. I know that AIDS is not caused by
sex. It is not the result of my sexuality or punishment for being gay, or black, or young, or female,
or anything. I know and affirm that I am a child
of God.

Being a child of God, I am godlike. I am divine.
And I know that when I smile on myself, all the
stars in heaven smile on me too.

I love myself just the way I am.

To heal is to touch with love that which
we previously touched with fear.
— Stephen Levine

How often, to avoid painful memories or feelings, have we tried to find escape in the numbing safety of alcohol, other drugs, sex, or food? When we were using we were seldom conscious of what set us off. Perhaps we tapped into our grief, our rage, or some memory — some storehouse of pain.

Whatever it was, we reacted out of fear of pain. Our system went into action to make sure we avoided having our feelings. It was a survival technique that served us well. But somewhere along the line, our addictions and survival techniques stopped working for us.

Now, with the loving support of our friends, a Twelve Step program, and a Higher Power, we can face our fears without the aid of food, chemicals, or sex. Now, when we hurt, we can give ourselves love, and we can ask for help from others. Maybe we need someone to sit and listen. Maybe we need to be touched or held.

We no longer need to act out of fear.

Today I am willing to be sad, angry, joyful, rageful, or filled with grief. I will love all my emotions. I know that I can ask for help whenever I need it.

February

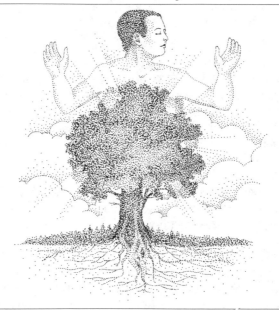

I imagine that I am a tree. Down through the base of my spine I send my roots deep and wide into the earth. I send my branches to the sky. I am a growing, breathing vital spiritual human being.

*Let My worship be in the heart that
rejoices, for behold — all acts of love and
pleasure are My rituals.*
— The Star Goddess from the Spiral Dance

Many of us grew up in an atmosphere of guilt
and shame. We were taught early on that our feelings were somehow not okay. We stopped expressing our emotions, stopped touching others, and little
by little we shut down.

We were told our sexual feelings were especially
bad and could get us into big trouble. We felt guilty.
Some of us spent years denying this. No, no, we
protested, we were liberated and free. But in
actuality we were numb from alcohol and other
drugs, or acting out with compulsive sex.

Now we are learning how to really get rid of, not
just deny, all the old baggage we've been carrying
around. We are learning that all the denied feelings from the past must surface: the anger, the
frustration, and the grief.

Releasing old emotions allows us to finally move
on and reclaim our natural, sexual, emotional,
innocent, human selves.

---

*I am a beautiful child of the universe. I rejoice in my
sexuality. I claim my rich humanity. I am happy,
joyous, free.*

When we inhale, the air comes into the inner world. When we exhale, the air goes out to the outer world. The inner world is limitless, and the outer world is also limitless. We say "inner world" or "outer world," but actually there is just one whole world.
      — *Zen Mind Beginner's Mind*

Those of us fighting AIDS can easily become preoccupied with keeping up with all the latest news. Just managing our treatments can demand most of our time. We look for tools to help keep ourselves and people we love alive and well: medicine, meditation, support groups. In all the activity, it's easy to forget a powerful healing tool — breathing. When we bring our attention to our breath, we let go of stress and give our immune system the opportunity it needs to heal.

This is not to say that all the other work we do isn't important. It is. But it can be much more useful when we are balanced and peaceful. Attention to our breath immediately brings awareness of harmony.

I breathe in, I am filled with love. I breathe out, I extend love. I am empty. I am full. I am emptiness. I am fullness.

. . . for behold, the kingdom of God is within you.

— *Luke 17:21*

Many of us left the religion of our childhood long ago. Some of us suffered the disapproval of a church that told us because of our sexual preference we were inherently sinful. So we rejected religion and, with it, we may have rejected our own spirituality.

Some of us found that the longer we used alcohol, other drugs, and sex, or pursued material possessions, the more distant and cut off we became from our spirituality. The emptiness inside kept needing to be filled and we kept looking for something to fill it. When we acquired what we thought would make us happy, it didn't. Confused and disappointed, we turned our attention to something else.

Now, recovery and the challenge of AIDS is teaching us how to reclaim our spiritual selves. When we feel empty or sad, confused or afraid, we know that we can go inside for comfort. There we remember that we are one with the world. We are everything, we have everything, we are complete and whole now, in this moment.

My heart is filled with love. I have everything. I am everything. I am at peace.

People who know I have AIDS see me and, because I look fine, they don't know what to talk about. Much of this disease is hidden.
— *Keith Gann, person with AIDS*

For some of us, AIDS means continual medical care. But for many of us, AIDS is about living day after day much like everyone else. We don't look different.

Or maybe we don't even have an AIDS diagnosis. We just tested positive or are in a high risk group. Maybe we're affected by AIDS because of all the people around us who are affected by AIDS. Regardless of our health status, AIDS can powerfully affect our feelings.

It's important not to deny or stuff our feelings. When we're angry, or afraid, or sad, we need to make a special effort to open up and talk. When everything is going well, we need support too. We need support for being well, for feeling good, for being okay. We need to make a special effort to get positive support and encouragement for being a well person affected by AIDS.

I ask for and deserve love and attention no matter what the state of my health. I deserve love and attention regardless of whether I have a diagnosis or not.

Visualize yourself standing before a gate-
way on a hilltop. Your entire life lies
out behind you and below. Before you step
through, pause and review the past: the
learning and the joys, the victories and
the sorrows — everything it took to bring
you here.

— The Book of Runes

Sometimes, to move forward we must look at where we've been. When we feel frustrated, blocked, or anxious, it may be because we need to deal with some old unfinished business. Often, these old hurts, painful memories, or shameful experiences are secrets we've never told anyone. While they remain secret they have the power to disrupt our lives.

The Twelve Step program teaches us how to make peace with the past. We are encouraged to write down our story, all of it, and then we are asked to tell it, including all our secrets, to someone we trust. Once we do, our past begins to lose its ability to control us. We take a big step toward being free of old hurts, wounds, injustices. And in the process we begin to forgive ourselves and others.

All that's required is willingness and honesty.

Today I will take time to review my past. I will begin to tell my story, including all my secrets.

*I am willing to release the pattern in me
that is creating this condition.*
— *Louise Hay*

When we want to make big life changes such as becoming sober, smoke-free, or physically fit, FEAR moves in. "It will hurt too much. You won't be able to handle the anxiety and the pain. You won't have any friends . . . ."

If that doesn't work, FEAR asks PANIC for help and that usually takes care of it. We light up, have a drink, shoot up, or go to the refrigerator. FEAR keeps us focused on the condition we want to change and diverts our attention from the pattern that keeps us stuck in the first place. Our habits are only symptoms of self-defeating patterns and belief systems. To get rid of the symptoms we have to be willing to get rid of the patterns. Letting go of our self-defeating beliefs and behavior means letting go of who we think we are and finding out who we really are. It means being willing to stand for a while feeling confused and naked.

Luckily, all it takes is a little willingness, just a small yes that says, "I'm willing to give up the old and see what the world has in store for me."

Today I am willing to let my ego relax and let my higher self take control.

It is the state of deep, constant Love and abiding caringness for all things that you seek. . . . Please give all due heart and mind to the need for finding that state of Love within your own being.
— *Bartholomew*

AIDS can make us desperate to find a lover. We're in a hurry to find someone to satisfy our craving for love, someone to fill that empty place. Or we look for other things like the perfect apartment, more money, new clothes.

What we want is peace. We want to be centered, and filled with love for ourselves and for everyone we meet. But we secretly believe we lack certain things essential to peace and serenity, so we must wait until we get what we are missing.

The truth is we have everything we need to be at perfect peace now. This instant. We need to want it now. And we need to look inside to find it. When we expect other people and material things to make us happy, we will always be disappointed. There is a place inside us, however, that is always in perfect peace.

I will stop my craving for outside fixes and look inside for what I need. As I breathe in and out, I find the abiding source of love.

Acceptance is the activity of love.
— *Samuel Kirshmer*

When we deny the truth about ourselves, we invest our problems with a whole lot of energy. We rationalize our character defects with statements like, "I'm not intolerant, I'm just sensitive." It takes a lot of energy to keep up our rationalizations and clever denials. Acceptance frees that energy and lets us get on with living.

Acceptance isn't resignation. We can accept some aspect of ourselves without being resigned to it. By accepting where we are we make change possible.

Acceptance of AIDS empties the disease of much of its power. Accepting our fear, anger, and resentment helps us get beyond the point of resistance to a gentler place of healing and letting go. Acceptance sends a message to the little child inside us that says, "However you feel is totally okay with me. I love you just the way you are."

And once we accept our own humanness, it's easier to accept other people too. Just the way they are.

Today I will practice sending myself messages of total acceptance. Whatever comes up, I will be gentle and accepting.

*One does not have to stand against
the gale.
One yields and becomes part of the wind.*
— *Emmanuel*

Like the willow tree that bends with the wind,
we show our strength when we surrender, yield,
and become part of the wind. In the same way, we
become free when we turn our will over to the care
of God.

Many of us are so tense from fighting against the
wind that we don't even know it. Only when we
relax a little do we sense the need to relax a lot,
the need to go limp and surrender.

Fear holds us back. We are afraid that we will
disappear or lose our identity. We are afraid that
God's will for us will be alien and unpleasant.

But when we listen to that small voice inside, we
are tuning into the will of God. The more we are
true to ourselves, the more we act in harmony with
the universe. We don't have to fight the wind; we
are the wind.

---

*I relax all tension and tightness from trying to make
it happen, from trying to resist my true nature. I know
that I am one with the wind. I relax and let go.*

The only thing that is required for healing is a lack of fear. The fearful are not healed, and cannot heal. This does not mean the conflict must be gone forever from your mind to heal . . . but it does mean, if only for an instant, you love without attack. An instant is sufficient. Miracles wait not on time.

— *A Course in Miracles*

Again and again we discover fear hiding behind other emotions. We find fear causing us to use old behaviors, to act out old hurts. Behind our fear is the belief that we can be attacked and hurt. This is like the fear of children who can't count on their parents to protect them.

Our healing begins when we realize that we are not children anymore. Then, instead of seeing people as powerful potential attackers, we see others as our brothers and sisters.

Finally, we stop acting out of fear; we stop attacking ourselves; we stop the constant criticism, and every once in a while, just for a moment, we sigh deeply and simply love ourselves. What rest in that instant. What calm certainty of peace.

I believe in miracles. I am not afraid. I trust the world. I love myself.

Doctors spend their time looking for the symptoms of illness, rarely acknowledging that illness is itself a symptom.
— Margo Adair

When we get ill, our bodies are saying we're out of sync. Either our behavior needs changing, our attitudes, our environment, or a combination of all three. If we accept our illness as a gift — a messenger carrying important information — we can begin to change the real problems. First we must listen. By careful listening, those of us affected by AIDS are learning a lot about ourselves.

AIDS may also be a messenger for an entire society that is out of balance. If so, those of us learning our individual lessons about AIDS can help the world learn the lessons it needs to learn in order to heal the planet.

As we imagine ourselves healed, we can also "image" a healed planet. As we learn to send light, energy, and love to ourselves and to each other, we can also send love to our Mother, the earth.

Today I will listen to the messages my body sends me. I will treat my disease and not just my symptoms. Today I will send loving energy to my body and to my Mother, the earth.

We had to deny our feelings in our trau-
matic childhoods; we thus became es-
tranged from all our feelings, and lost the
ability to recognize and express them.
— *From "The Problem" published*
by Adult Children of Alcoholics

We certainly don't have to be from alcoholic
families to have had traumatic childhoods. Many
of us have blocked so much of that early pain that
we scarcely remember being children.

It's likely, however, that it wasn't safe or okay to
express our feelings. Now as adults, we have a very
limited vocabulary for our feelings. Maybe we have
one emotion, such as anger or shame, that covers
for all of them.

We can't go back and relive our childhoods, but
we can begin to re-parent ourselves. We can treat
that delicate, feeling part of ourselves with gentleness and caring. As we do, we become more aware
of our feelings. We learn that we have a rainbow
of emotions to choose from. Every time we feel one
of the colors in the rainbow we become more alive
and real.

I will sit quietly today and pay attention to what I am
feeling. I will experience the feeling even if I don't yet
know its name.

The more we freely choose to operate within our present bodily limits, the more spiritually unlimited we become.
— Dr. Aaron Flickstein

Many of us spent years abusing our bodies with alcohol and other drugs, compulsive sex, food, cigarettes, and negative emotions. For a while, our bodies seemed to take it. The effects took awhile to show.

Now we are learning that there are consequences for what we put into and do to our bodies. We are learning that our bodies have limits and needs. For example, we all need exercise and sleep, though in slightly different amounts. As we listen and pay attention, we begin to discover our personal limits. We find that certain foods and activities are outside our limits even if they are fine for other people.

When we violate our limits, we clog up and begin to feel cut off again, alienated, addicted. When we honor our limits, we become open and clear channels and allow the spirit of the universe to flow through us.

I honor and respect my limits. I open myself to the unlimited vastness of space and spirit.

Purpose is a fixed horizon that we never reach but that gives us a general direction in life. Goals are the passing landmarks that tell us we are indeed moving. . . . Goals commit us to life.
— Tom O'Connor, person with ARC

AIDS has our attention. Unfortunately, for some of us it has all our attention. That's all we can see on the horizon. But that's a choice. We can choose to focus only on AIDS or we can choose to focus on dreams and goals separate from AIDS. We all need to see that what we focus on is our choice. If we choose to focus on the positive lessons AIDS can teach us, we may discover dreams and goals we'd like to work toward.

What are my goals? Can I write them down? What have I been focusing on? Have I been exercising my right to choose, or have I been going along with what newspapers and television tell me to focus on?

Are my goals reachable? Are they too easy and not challenging? What do I really want to be? How do I really want to live my life? What did I want to be when I was a child? What are my dreams?

Today I get to think about my life's purpose. I know that I always have choices. I will choose a purpose and goals that ring true in my heart.

I have learned that I deserve to give myself
all the care and love I give others.
— *Tom Agar*

AIDS is teaching us how to love, nurture, and support each other. Sometimes the challenge seems overwhelming. We wonder if there just isn't too much pain, hurt, and fear.

Many of us are either professional caregivers or primary caregivers to loved ones. We give and give. Too often we lose focus and only later realize, "Oh, I'm still here!" We realize that we've been gone somewhere, lost in the lives of others.

That's when the Twelve Step program and our friends can gently bring us back to our center, to what the yogis call the *hara*, the second *chakra*, a place just below our navel. We can pull in our scattered energy, and root ourselves in the earth like a tree.

Because, our first job is to love ourselves. If we do that well enough we will be able to spread love wherever we go.

Today I will place my name at the top of the list of people deserving my special love. I will attend to those things that are important to my well-being. I will nourish myself.

How could anyone ever, ever not want the kind of love I have to offer? It's preposterous.
— Robert Keene, person with AIDS

Doubt. Anxiety. Fear of rejection. Oh, how those low opinions we have of ourselves hold us back from acting courageously, boldly. We even doubt the value and the quality of the love we have to offer.

Each one of us has special talents and abilities and a unique way of being in this world. When we find ourselves doubting our value, we need to listen to what the voice inside us is saying. Is it being critical and judgmental? Where did it learn to speak the way it does?

To change negative thoughts about ourselves we have to recognize them and experience any feelings associated with them. And then we need to change our thoughts. We need to replace our old beliefs with new affirmations such as: I am a great lover. I am a healer. I am filled with spirit. Everyone wants the kind of love I have to offer.

Today I affirm aloud. I am wonderfully loving. I heal the world with my love.

Having what is called insight,
A good man, before he can help a
   bad man,
Finds in himself the matter with the
   bad man.
That is the heart of it.
                              — *Lao Tsu*

Some people push our buttons, irritate us, and get under our skin. No matter what we do, they keep our attention. Though we don't like this feeling, it's so hard not to be critical.

That is, until we see that person as ourselves. When we do, we realize that the people who irritate us are simply mirroring characteristics that we have and don't want to look at. Likewise, the people who we're most attracted to are also mirroring us. We have those qualities too.

There's nothing we can do about the other person. We can, however, attend to what's really bothering us — our own fears and character defects. We can be loving, attentive, forgiving, and kind to ourselves. Then it's easier to be loving to others.

Today I will be thankful for all the people placed in my life. They hold up mirrors. I will look into the mirrors, notice what needs changing, and appreciate what is beautiful.

The fundamental problem most patients have is an inability to love themselves, having been unloved by others during some crucial part of their lives.

— Bernie Siegel

Most of us have to go way back in our lives to remember a time when we felt sure of ourselves and our places in the world. Some of us can't recall any time when we didn't feel somehow unacceptable. We were taught right away that our natural feelings weren't okay with mother or father. And if they wouldn't accept us just the way we were, nobody would.

The shame caused by this lack of acceptance can make us sick. The first step to healing and recovery is learning to love ourselves the way we are. Every little act of self-acceptance and self-love allows us to relax a bit more, to let down our defenses, to show people who we are. And little by little we learn to cry. We learn to experience our emotions. We learn to trust ourselves and each other.

I am learning all the wonderful skills of self-love. Every positive action I take proves that I am lovable.

*We all know it all. We know everything
— all the connections.*
  — Tony Petzel, person with AIDS

It's difficult to lift the veils that keep our consciousness clouded and confused. But there is a part of all of us that is connected to deep knowing, a place where our memory is ancient and true, a place where we are as we are meant to be.

Perhaps our job in this lifetime is to find our way back to that place. Lessons are given to us to help us remember who we are. The path back home is our quest, our search for our holy grail.

Little by little, we realize that we already are who we want to be. We have an inkling of an idea that we already know what we need to know, and we begin to remember and understand that we are connected to every living thing.

AIDS is helping many of us lift concealing veils and let go of unnecessary baggage. AIDS can help us find our way home to healing, safety, knowing, and connectedness.

---

*I have everything. I know everything. I am at peace.
I am connected through every cell of my body to mother
earth, to father sun, and to all the stars in heaven.*

The Soul of man
Resembleth water:
From heaven it cometh,
To heaven it soareth . . .
Changing ever.
— *Goethe*

We don't need to wait for another lifetime to
have a transformation. We need only connect ourselves with the image of water, which cleans, heals,
and transforms. Our bodies are, after all, mostly
water, and the cleansing image of water can make
us feel reborn.

Consider the unending transformation of water
as it travels from rain, to ocean, to evaporation, to
clouds, to rain, to rivers and streams, to us, through
us, to oceans, clouds, to rain, from water to ice, from
ice to steam.

As we become one with water and send our attention upward to the heavens and downward into
rivers and streams, we follow the path of water and
its transformation. We cleanse our souls and heal
our bodies. We die and are reborn.

Every contact with water can be a chance to connect to this mystery.

Water is holy. By water I am healed and made clean.

I am larger, better than I thought. I did not know I held so much goodness.
— Walt Whitman

What is my self-image? How big am I? How big am I in relation to other people, friends, family, doctors, employers, authority figures? If I were to draw a picture of myself next to all these people what would I look like?

Those of us who grew up in dysfunctional families probably see ourselves child-sized. Although to the world we look like adults, inside we feel like teenagers or children, small and afraid.

The truth is, we are adults, larger and better than we thought. And we have a right to take up adult-sized space. We have a right to command adult attention. We have the adult ability to protect ourselves.

Whenever we start to feel child-sized we can draw another picture. We can draw ourselves adult-sized with our arms around the shoulders of a little child, protectively comforting that part of us that is afraid.

I am big and strong and good. I have a right to take up space. The little child inside me feels safe and secure.

Man can only receive what he sees himself receiving.
— *Florence Scovel Shinn*

How does it feel to be vibrantly healthy? How do I respond when the universe gives me the gift of glorious health?

Calmly visualizing ourselves in states of perfect well-being may be the most important healing step we can take. Sometimes, though, when we relax, close our eyes and picture ourselves, we are blocked. We hear voices or see images of people who long ago told us we couldn't or wouldn't or didn't deserve to be everything we wanted to be. Now we can tell those voices they are wrong and tell them to leave. As we let go of the voices that aren't ours we can reclaim the feelings that are. We become more whole, more of who we truly are.

As we return to the visualization, we move past the place of resistance and imagine ourselves more happy, more joyous, and more free than we thought any person could be.

I see myself receiving magnificent, brilliantly glowing gifts from the universe. Gifts of health, love, and perfect self-expression. I am filled with joy.

It's not as though one day you have an exchange and get sick. We all have a long history of immuno suppressive behavior that leads up to the present.
— Bill Kummer, person with ARC

Recovery (from AIDS, alcoholism, or drug addiction) gives us the opportunity to tell the truth about who we are, the whole story, everything that brought us to where we are today. For many of us, being honest about our childhoods and adulthoods is a painful and new experience.

But only when we get honest do we begin to see the patterns, the behaviors, and situations that keep repeating themselves in our relationships, jobs, illnesses, accidents, and sexual relations.

Honesty helps us break the patterns, learn the lessons, bless the past, and let it go.

It's a great relief — mentally, emotionally, and physically — to finally tell the story about where we've been.

Today I pray for the courage to honestly look at my past and the willingness to admit to myself and to others the truth about my life.

*When the past has taught us that we have
more within us than we have ever used,
our prayer is a cry to the divine to come
to us and fill us with its power.*
— Rudolph Steiner

When finally we honestly look at our lives, we
are usually confronted with a painful reality. We
don't measure up to our ideals or to that vague
sense of unlimited potential that we know is our
true self.

How do we tap that deep well of possibility? How
do we reach in to become as creative, loving, intense,
and expansive as we intuitively know we can be?
Many of us tried to reach that place with alcohol,
other drugs, and sometimes with sex. Or, we tried
to ignore the reality of our lives by drowning it out
in a sea of numbness.

Prayer that cries out from an honest look at our
past is a prayer for help, a prayer for power. Our
addictions have failed us. When finally we accept
our humanness without shame or guilt, and pray
for help, help comes. And sooner or later, we realize
that we are more wonderful than we ever imagined.

---

*Today I will honestly look at my life and humbly ask
for divine power to flow through me, so that I may
manifest my true self.*

Every moment we can choose our point of view. We can choose to see AIDS as a grim crisis for humanity or as an extraordinary opportunity, individually and collectively, to move forward.

— Christopher Spence

Every moment we choose our point of view. This moment we can choose to be grateful for the experience of AIDS. We can recognize AIDS as a teacher. We can ask for help to learn its lessons about our spiritual and loving natures.

In the days before AIDS, many of us didn't know how to express our love for each other or how to ask for what we needed. Instead, we tried to fill the emptiness inside and soothe our aching hearts with sex, alcohol, drugs, or all three. When we were done, we still felt empty.

Now we are learning about living in a loving community. Each step we take out of isolation, out of addiction, out of our old behavior, is a major achievement, a healing action.

I choose my point of view. AIDS is an outrageous opportunity for me and for all of us. I choose to let the experience of AIDS help me move forward.

On my way to my lover's funeral, my mother said, "You've got to be strong. His parents won't be able to deal with a crying gay lover." So I was strong.

— John

All of us have oceans of grief dammed up inside. Behind our anger and rage is a deep, painful sadness. Behind our eyes are tears ready to be shed, needing to be released.

It's important that each of us creates a safe place where we can weep, rage, wail, and cry. Where there are support groups and bereavement groups, we can take advantage of them. We can also share our sadness with special friends or in organized religious settings. There are also times when we need to be alone with our sadness.

The important thing is that we take the time to grieve. Expressing our grief opens a space around our heart and gives us room to breathe. We become more open to the world around us, and are able to live more fully in the present.

I am safe, secure, and protected. I am willing to grieve. Today I will open a place in my heart that has been closed off.

When people asked, I used to tell them how sick I was. The more I talked about being sick, the worse I got. Finally I started saying, "I'm getting better." It took a while, but then I started to feel better too.
— *Michael Hirsch, person with AIDS*

Our words point us in the direction we go. It's very important to choose them carefully. If we constantly talk about feeling bad, we invest our illnesses with a lot of power. Energy is directed through our words and our thoughts. The universe supports us negatively or positively.

Of course we need to talk honestly about our health and our emotional state. However, when we talk about where we are or how we feel, we can also add a positive word or thought about where we want to go.

Our words are our tools. They are at work, building our future, whether we are conscious of it or not. What words do we use? What are we saying to ourselves and to others? What do our friends and the people around us say? Is it positive?

My words make magic. They help me heal and grow and transform. Today I use my words to help me heal and to establish my power.

Dream of your brother's kindnesses instead
of dwelling in your dreams of his mistakes.
Select his thoughtfulness to dream about
instead of counting up the hurts he gave.
— *A Course in Miracles*

Resentments are nasty little ideas that cling to the insides of our minds and won't let go. Just when we think they're gone, they pop up and cloud our minds with anger and hurt.

Many times our hurts are real. But even justified resentment is painful to live with. The Twelve Step program and other spiritual programs offer us help. They help us see the people we're afraid of or angry with are really very much like us. Like us, they're trying to find their way and often make mistakes in the process.

As soon as we're able to forgive others, we can begin to look at our own behavior and see where we might be able to change. The minute our focus returns to ourselves, our power returns too. This power allows us to stop being helpless victims and start being powerful actors able to forgive others and ourselves.

I am grateful for all the people in my life. I forgive myself and all others who I feel may ever have harmed me.

Only when you have no thing in your mind
and no mind in things are you vacant and
spiritual, empty and marvelous.
  — The Gospel According to Zen

We can all take time to meditate today. We can sit on pillows on the floor, or sit upright in a straight-backed chair, or lie on the floor with our head slightly raised. The main thing is that we relax our bodies and let all tension and anxiety go, muscle after muscle, from head to toe.

Peace and harmony are more than ideas. They are feelings that can happen to us. All we need to do is ready ourselves to receive them. Meditation is a good way to practice readiness. The more we practice the easier it is to receive.

Today I will practice readiness. I will meditate. I will let the busyness of the world slip away. I will be at ease.

March

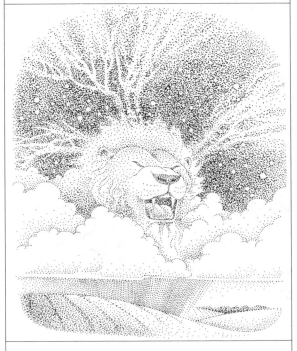

Today I will roar like an angry lion. I will let my rage out into the universe in ways that are totally harmonious for everyone concerned.

Gravity is the root of grace,
The mainstay of all speed.
A traveler of true means, whatever the
day's pace,
Remembers the provision van.
                                            — *Lao Tsu*

Sometimes we get ahead of ourselves. We produce more stress than we can handle in a healthy way.

We get too busy to meditate. We get too busy to take a walk with a friend, write in our journal, or read. We miss meetings or meals or stop going to the gym. We get too far ahead of our spiritual provision van.

The result is relapse. Oh, we may not actually slip or go back into the hospital, but we begin to have a spiritual relapse. Then, our bodies let us know something is wrong. And if we pay attention to all the little warning signals along the way, we won't need a major catastrophe. We'll remember what's important, what's first. We'll remember our program — what keeps us rested and relaxed, healthy and vital. We'll respect and honor our spiritual provision van.

Today I will put first things first. I will stay close to what keeps me connected, physically, and spiritually. I will honor and respect myself.

I love myself just the way I am,
there's nothing I need to change
I'll always be the perfect me,
there's nothing to rearrange
— Jai Josefs

We tell ourselves, I'll love myself after . . . I lose twenty pounds, gain twenty pounds, get rid of these lesions, beat this disease. . . . Now let's try it again from the top: I love myself just the way I am. There's nothing I need to change.

This is part of the first verse to a wonderful song about unconditional love. It's a good verse to repeat again and again, aloud, looking into the mirror, looking into our own eyes, smiling at ourselves.

If we have trouble looking in the mirror and being kind, maybe we need to stay with the feelings that surface when we look in the mirror and then try to remember when it was that we stopped feeling good about ourselves. Who told us we weren't good enough?

Then, throughout the day, we need to treat ourselves as we would treat someone we were madly in love with — surprise gifts, spontaneous hugs, the works.

I love myself just the way I am.

Disease is undeveloped health.
— Ann Wigmore

Modern western medicine often concentrates on illness, not wellness. Giant medical clinics and massive research facilities employ thousands of doctors and scientists to study disease.

No wonder we tend to ignore our bodies most of the time and then, when ill, focus on the disease. But we have a choice. We can see illness as a curse, or we can see illness as the path our bodies are taking us to health. We can be angry with our bodies for failing us, or we can listen to what our bodies are trying to tell us.

We need to make sure we're making the choice that is right for us. We need to make sure we aren't being negatively pressured by the huge weight of the existing medical establishment. Because we *do* have the option to focus on our health, not just our disease. We *can* see illness as our body's way of telling us what we need to do now to be physically, emotionally, and spiritually healthy.

I choose health and healing. My illnesses are like sign-posts that keep me moving in the right direction.

*. . . you just can't heal the physical body
without coming to grips with the pattern
that created the symptoms of your disease
in the first place.*
— Irene Smith

Illnesses don't just happen; they happen to us.
Along the way we each acquired certain beliefs,
attitudes, and behaviors that fit together and
created a pattern — an individual way of being. Just
as many of us who are alcoholics realize "the bottle
was only a symptom," many of us realize AIDS is
only a symptom, a symptom of the patterns that
hold us locked in low self-esteem, lack of love,
and loneliness.

We stay locked in the prisons of those patterns
until we take an honest look at our lives. We take
time to reflect. We ask our friends to help, and
sometimes we ask for professional help. We begin
to see where we're out of balance, where our beliefs
need changing. We begin to replace old patterns
with new immune-enhancing patterns.

*What are the patterns in my life that keep me trapped,
unable to move freely? Please help me find and release
all old beliefs, attitudes, and habits that keep me in
a state of dis-ease.*

A mirror not covered with dust is clear and bright. The mind should be like this. When what beclouds it passes away, its brightness appears. Happiness must not be sought for; when what disturbs passes away, happiness comes of itself.
— *The Gospel According to Zen*

"Have I done enough? . . . What should I do next? . . . Where will I get the money? . . . What if they cancel my insurance?" Grinding our teeth in fear of the future, certain that mistakes and patterns of our past would catch up with us, we wait for the other shoe to drop.

Always the answer is the same — be here now. Let the thoughts that cloud your mind pass away. They are just thoughts. Don't judge yourself for having them. Just notice them and let them drift away. Without attention they lose their power.

When we attempt to live one day at a time, we experience serenity. We learn about grace. We learn that each moment is new.

I sit quietly and allow my thoughts to pass. I imagine that I am a calm lake. I allow disturbing thoughts to drift away like clouds across the sky. I allow comfort and peace to surround and penetrate my body.

A Always
I In
D Divine
S Safety
  — *slogan from a Healing Circle button*

What a lovely alternative to the prevailing attitude that equates AIDS with fear. AIDS seems to foster fear. But then, so does reading a newspaper. And whether we're worried about our health or the condition of the planet, fear can paralyze us.

Behind the fear of AIDS is a belief that we are helplessly unprotected in a dangerous, unpredictable world. Most of the media and the medical community promote this belief with statements or phrases such as, "if you get AIDS you'll die," and "the deadly AIDS virus." But a belief is just a thought we're in the habit of thinking. We can change our thoughts. Instead of thinking about our aloneness, we can think about our at-one-ness. We can think about our unity and connection with all living things.

The more we think about being one with the power and love of the universe, the more our fear begins to be replaced with faith, and we acquire new habits of thinking that serve us better.

I am always in divine safety. I am protected and cared for.

*My body has been talking to me for years.
I just have to learn to listen.*

— Bob

Our bodies are great communicators. Sometimes, though, listening to our body is like listening to a dolphin. We know it's intelligent, but we can't quite make out what it's saying.

After a time, we begin to learn what certain messages mean. Like, "I feel a cold coming on, it's time to slow down." The more we pay attention, the more respectful we become of this incredible intelligence we have. We realize how important it is to learn the language of our body.

We also know that when we don't listen to the whispered messages, we get louder ones until we do pay attention. Getting a telegram from our body means we're connected, mind, body, and spirit.

That's why with AIDS or any illness, the point is to discover what the message is and be grateful for the lesson, not angry with the messenger.

I listen to my body. I pay attention to my pain and my fear and I listen. I am grateful for the information and send love to my body, the messenger.

Today I will make no decisions by myself.
  — A Course in Miracles

Instead, I will ask my inner knowing, my intuitive self, the God within, for direction. I will sit quietly and listen. I will imagine the kind of day I want: peaceful and productive, or exciting and stimulating. I will pause and ask how I want to feel today, what I want the day to be like. I will envision that kind of day and know that if I make no decisions by myself, that kind of day will be given to me.

When I take back control and make all the decisions by myself, when I worry and fret about whether I've made the right choice or not, I'm back to being separate, isolated, fearful, and alone again.

Instead, I will make no decisions by myself today. I will call a friend, my sponsor, a buddy, or all three just to talk about me. And I will consult my spirit guides and my Higher Power, because today I will make no decisions by myself.

I am part of a divine magical mystery team. We make our decisions together.

thymos (Greek): courage, vitality, spirit.

The thymus gland is the organ of courage. It is the basis for the dynamic of vital self-affirmation as the center of our immune system. The thymus gland is our vital center.

— Paul Lee

Located just behind the breast bone near our heart is our thymus, the most important endocrine gland in our immune system.

The energy associated with this gland is love — giving, receiving, expanding love. Opening our chest — our heart center — and expanding our awareness to accept more love, makes us more vital and alive.

Positive affirmations and the willingness to give and receive love helps activate our immune system and gives us the courage to be. This wonderful connection between our body, our mind, and our spirit is real and immediate. It is worth meditating on.

I gratefully acknowledge my amazing thymus gland. I open a space in my heart for it to flourish and thrive. I open my heart and accept the loving energy of the universe. I am vital and alive.

When you do not realize that you are one with the river, or one with the universe, you have fear. Whether it is separated into drops or not, water is water. Our life and death are the same thing. When we realize this thing we have no fear of death anymore, and we have no actual difficulty in our life.

— *Shunryu Suzuki*

When we are afraid, we have forgotten who we are. When we forget who we really are, we feel small, alone, and vulnerable. Like a drop of water.

Just as water doesn't stop being water once it's part of the river, we don't stop being part of the universe once we die. We are composed of the same elements that surround us. That is the reality. The illusion is the little ego, the public persona, the mask we hide behind.

The minute we forget who we are, fear creeps up again and limits our beliefs about who we are and what we can accomplish. When we remember we are the universe, all things are possible and we lose our fears.

I am one with the universe. I am constantly changing and evolving. I am not afraid. I always remember who I am.

I forgive myself for having believed for so long that . . . I was never good enough to have, get, be what I wanted.
— Ceanne DeRohan

We all carry judgments about ourselves that need to be released. One of the biggest judgments we make is based on guilt. Many of us heard society judging us. We decided we didn't deserve a good life because we're gay, black, Hispanic, female, or just different. We felt guilty for being the way we are. We internalized society's hate and learned to hate ourselves.

The way out of these negative judgments is through forgiveness. We need to forgive ourselves for holding guilt and judgment; we need to accept all the old feelings of hurt associated with low self-esteem, sexual guilt, and feelings of inadequacy. This process of forgiveness allows us to experience the pain caused by these judgments, pain that we've been running from for a long time. Experiencing the feeling instead of running from it is true release, real letting go.

I forgive myself for all past judgments against myself. I now affirm that I am a beautiful, creative child of God. I deserve all good things.

*Peace of mind sends the body a "live"
message, while depression, fear, and
unresolved conflict give it a "die" message.*
— Bernie Siegel

People who study the effects of the mind on
healing are learning that attitude is important
to healing. We can't deny this fact anymore. Our
state of mind has a lot to do with our state of health.
It is up to us to learn to live in peace.

Unresolved conflict, internalized anger, and fear
combine to suppress our immune system. Stress
keeps us sick. So how do we resolve these feelings?
Most of us need help from friends, sponsors, coun-
selors, support groups, and help from our spiritual
source, from a Higher Power.

Accepting help requires willingness. And even if
we can't be totally willing, we can be willing to
be willing. It doesn't take much to let miracles
happen. The smallest bit of willingness is the
beginning of faith.

*I am at peace. I now willingly allow great miracles
to happen in my life.*

The only way to speak the truth is to speak lovingly.

— *Thoreau*

Sometimes the truth is painful. It hurts to look at our lives and discover that the reality of who we are doesn't match our ideals or dreams. Yet only when we're honest with ourselves do we move forward.

However, if we tell ourselves the "painful truth" in a critical and blaming way we throw all the benefits of honesty out the window. Constant criticism and judgment don't help us move forward; they just keep us stuck in shame. So when we decide to be honest we need to be forgiving too.

Whenever that harsh, critical voice starts yapping inside our heads, we know it's time to stop, calm ourselves, and gently ask the voice to be quiet and leave. We also know it's time to be extra kind and gentle with ourselves. It's time to tell the little child inside that everything is okay and that we love him or her very much.

I leave all criticism and blame behind. I always counsel myself in a loving, accepting voice. The truth is easy to hear.

*As one of Thomas Merton's monks has it,
"Go into your cell and your cell will teach
you everything there is to know." Your cell.
Your self.*

— Akshara Noor

We have many ways to avoid being alone. We read. We smoke cigarettes, and watch TV. We stay busy. We keep on the move, running from ourselves. Some of us even run from one healing workshop to another looking for teachers. When we find them, they tell us to be still, meditate. But we continue to scurry about, ask questions, take notes, and buy more books that we think will tell us how to find peace.

Which is OK. It's part of the process. We each have a path to follow, and we must do it our own way. Because sooner or later, we stop smoking, turn off the TV, stay home, sit still, and listen.

We discover how much we love being alone with our self. And little by little we find that as we learn to be a good friend to our self, we also become better friends to other people. We are able to sit still and listen to them too.

Today I will stop my busyness for awhile and go into my cell and listen.

*Thy will be done this day! Today is a day
of completion; I give thanks for this perfect day, miracle shall follow miracle and
wonders shall never cease.*
— Florence Scovel Shinn

The quality of each day depends very much on
how we start it. Beginning with a powerful affirmation like the one above, points us in the right
direction. It helps us focus on the gift of today.

It's easy to say "live one day at a time," but it's
difficult to shake off fear, to stop the tapes that wind
and rewind in our minds, to not rehearse tomorrow's conflict, to not live in yesterday's hurts or
tomorrow's fears.

The only way we learn to live one day at a time
is by doing it — starting now. Always starting now.
When fears for the future arise we remember that
our lives are in the hands of a Higher Power. When
resentments surface we can ask for willingness to
be forgiving. When thoughts disturb us we can let
them pass like clouds on a summer day.

*I give thanks for this perfect day. I give thanks for
miracles already on their way. Today is given to me
to enjoy. Today is a magical, precious gift.*

Then, sighing, said the other, "Have thy will, I am the love that dare not speak its name."

— Lord Alfred Douglas

On October 11, 1987, more than 500,000 people marched in Washington, D.C., in support of civil rights for gay people. For one weekend, the city was gay. We were the majority. And having it this way for once helped many of us understand how deeply isolated, separate, and threatened we have felt.

Because many of our feelings and fears are brought on by real oppression, real violence, and real discrimination, we have developed a belief system that expects opposition and hatred. We expect to be discounted.

Now, AIDS is teaching us that we must be strong in our belief in ourselves and in our belief in unity. The more loving support we receive, the easier it is to walk in the world, tall and strong, clear that we belong.

Those of us who have felt the most alienated can teach the world about unity by stepping out of a system of alienation and becoming leaders in love.

I am not afraid of being who I am. When I am true to myself I am most united with you. Today I choose to live in unity. I will be a leader and teacher for love.

*Joining hands in the circle of abundance
    and love
We are blessed and we prosper wherever
    we turn
We receive what we want and we share
    what we can
Joining hands in the circle of abundance
    and love*
        — Joshua Leeds and Louise Hay

It's hard for some of us to ask for help and be willing to receive love and attention when we're feeling well. When we're sick, it's even harder. That's when all the old feelings of shame and guilt come racing back. We feel unacceptable and assume that others don't want us around.

That's when we need to get together with friends or go to support group meetings and tell people how we feel. By being honest about our feelings, we give others the chance to be honest too, and with a little help from our friends, we begin to replace the worn-out old tapes with new messages about love and acceptance.

Today I will talk about how I feel. I will ask for support. And I will make a special effort to reach out to my friends who are sick because I know they may be having a hard time asking for help.

By means of prayer we realize that the future is set before us by world wisdom. If we surrender ourselves to this feeling we produce something quite different than we do when we meet coming events with fear and anxiety.
— Rudolph Steiner

Certainly, logic doesn't support a belief that "the future is set before us by world wisdom." A glance at the headlines could easily provoke us to face the world with fear and anxiety. Often, only when we reach the end of our rope, only when we hit bottom from drinking, drugging, or AIDS, are we ready to try an approach that doesn't seem logical. Then we become willing to surrender to the situation and submit to the future. We open to another way of looking at the world. We begin to pray.

When we surrender and submit to the future, the world stops looking like a hopeless place. Fear becomes faith. Anxiety becomes serenity.

I look forward, with faith, to the future. I submit to a wisdom greater than my own. I am at peace.

You who are the source of all power
Whose rays illuminate the whole world,
Illuminate also my heart
So that it too can do your work.
— *The Book of Runes*

The power of this prayer is enhanced if, while saying it aloud, we visualize the sun's rays streaming toward the earth into our hearts and from our hearts into the world around us. All dark spaces lighten and our true self becomes clear and bright. Finally, we can see who we are.

The light that gives life to the world is available to us. All we need to do is open up the doors to our heart and let in the sunlight. Many of those doors are old and creaky and rusted shut. We may need help opening them. Inside are our secrets and hurts. We guard them carefully with shoulders hunched forward closed in around our heart. And we stay dark.

When we stand up straight, throw our shoulders back, lift our head and fill our lungs with air, we lighten our spirit. When we tell our secrets and talk about our fears and doubts, the doors swing open and the light shines in.

Today I will unlock locks and swing open doors that have kept my heart in darkness.

*We can learn to forgive ourselves for being
who we are, and to detach from what we
did not cause and cannot control.*
    — *from "The Solution"
    published by Adult Children
    of Alcoholics*

Next to, "I love you," the most important words
we need to hear from ourselves are, "I forgive you."
Standing in front of a mirror, looking into our own
eyes, we need to say these words over and over again.

I forgive you for being less than perfect. I forgive
you for being human. I forgive you for being compulsive and addictive. I forgive you for being intolerant and unforgiving. I love you and I forgive
you and I accept you just the way you are.

We need to acknowledge that life has been
difficult and that we're doing the best we can. And
in the spirit of love and acceptance, we need to
separate those things that we can change from those
things that we cannot. If we've been hanging on to
problems we can't control, we can bless them and
let them go.

*God grant me the serenity to accept the things I cannot
change, the courage to change the things I can, and
the wisdom to know the difference.*

I think one of the main reasons people with AIDS isolate and hide is shame.
— Ed, person with AIDS

Shame has been with us for a very long time. Even if we think we've worked through it, it's amazing what AIDS can do to reactivate shame.

Shame activates isolation. Afraid that we aren't good enough, we hide. We think if people find out who we are they'll leave. So, we avoid people or we avoid letting them know who we are.

AIDS is teaching us that people aren't shocked to learn we aren't perfect. Instead, when we allow them in, they love and accept us just the way we are. When that happens we start to recover. This is the miracle of recovery from AIDS, from alcoholism, from all those "shameful" diseases. Once we start telling the truth about who we are and how we really feel, we connect to other people more, not less.

As we examine our reflection in other people's eyes, we realize that we *are* worthwhile, beautiful, loveable. And little by little we lose our fear of people leaving us; we start looking forward to the new people who are entering our lives.

I love myself just the way I am. I am a child of God and have every right to be here.

My disease is one of the best things that has happened to me; it has pulled me out of a quietly desperate life toward one full of love and hope.
— Tom O'Connor, person with ARC

Those of us who have been addicted to alcohol or other drugs understand what it means to be quietly desperate. If we're lucky, we get desperate enough to ask for help. We somehow make a turn. We stop wanting to die and start wanting to live.

Now AIDS is forcing many more of us out of quiet desperation and into new relationships with others and with ourselves. We are making decisions to live. We are even deciding that we want to live well. Now.

We are letting go of unfulfilling jobs, outmoded attitudes, old behaviors, and people that keep us stuck in fear of the future and anger about the past. Little by little we are learning to live in the present, a day at a time.

I choose to live today as fully alive and present as I possibly can. I only have now, this moment. I want to fill it with love.

When you feel you can communicate only with other entities in physical bodies, you have cut yourself off from a powerful source of inner guidance.

— *Bartholomew*

The more we listen to our intuition, the more peaceful and serene we become. The closer our contact to our inner guide, or guardian angel, the safer we feel and the easier it is to make and carry out life-affirming decisions.

Even if we suspect we are only talking to ourselves, we're at least talking to our intuitive inner self, a part of ourselves that often gets ignored.

The point is, we don't have to believe, explain, or understand anything. It doesn't have to make sense. All we need to do is open our minds, suspend our judgment, and communicate — talk, ask questions, listen, feel, pay attention.

With an open mind and an open heart, I willingly receive help from places and beings I don't understand.

. . . parts of you are still in unfinished business.

— *Julius*

Every time we deny a feeling it becomes unfinished business. It doesn't go away, it waits to reappear. Sooner or later, unfinished business demands attention.

If we don't express feelings directly, they have a way of coming out sideways and unexpectedly: We say something mean or foolish, or we act inappropriately. The point is, we're not living in the present; we're acting out old emotions.

Unfinished business can also affect our health. Unfelt feelings can lodge in our muscles and tissues and nervous system and, if not expressed, can eventually make us sick.

Fortunately, we have an indicator of unfinished business — fear. When we notice the presence of fear, it's a good bet that behind it lies some injury or hurt that needs healing, some grief or anger that needs to be expressed.

I commit to reclaiming my total self from all unfinished business. I willingly express my feelings and open to expressing all old feelings that I once denied or suppressed.

Whatever you can do or dream you can do,
Begin it.
Boldness has genius and power and
  magic in it.
Begin it now.

— *Goethe*

Procrastination and fear are monster thieves. They eat up our lives. They steal hours, months, years. They leave us wondering where the time went and what happened to our dreams.

Sometimes our lethargy feels like a giant rock that can't be moved. But the rock is an illusion that weighs nothing and rolls away like a beach ball when we make the slightest effort.

That first action is incredibly powerful and reminds us of who we are. Every successive movement energizes us, especially when we are acting on our dreams. Even if all we do is pick up the phone, a pencil, or a brush.

Any action we take gives us power to take the next action and sets energy in motion all around us.

I move courageously in the direction of my dreams.
I live in the now. I am filled with energy and power.

In the moment of creation you were given incredible gifts; and one of the most important is the gift of sexuality.
— Mary Margaret Moore

Many of us know what it's like to use sex like a drug. We know what it's like to use sex to manipulate and control other people. And, at one time or another, most of us have felt shameful about our sexual feelings, about our bodies, or about our sexual history.

The world we grew up in didn't teach us how to honor and respect sexuality as a special gift. Instead, it taught us that sex was dirty. Those of us who are gay learned early on that we were fundamentally bad because of our sexuality.

But we are no longer children. All those ideas that imply our sexual energy is anything except a glorious gift from God can now be dumped. This instant.

From now on, we can vigilantly guard our sexuality from attack. This includes rejecting all propaganda that says AIDS is caused by sex.

We can begin to reclaim and re-create our sexual lives in joyous celebration and innocent delight.

I gratefully acknowledge that I am a sexual person. I honor and cherish my sexual self.

Childhood is the kingdom where nobody dies.
                    — *Edna St. Vincent Millay*

We don't live in the world of children anymore. All around us people have been dying. People our age. People like us. People too young to die. People who were our friends. People we used to talk to and eat with and make love to and hug.

We know that we don't live in the world of children anymore because our friends were here where we could touch them and now they're not. And we're adult enough not to look for them or expect them at any social gatherings. We also know we can forget about the hospital visit we were going to make, because our friend is dead.

Why is that? And why should our childhoods be over already? Who said? Who made it so? Why?

There is a part of us that needs to rage about what is happening to us. We could take a few good cues from children. They pound their fists, yell, and scream at injustice. We can do this too.

God bless my anger and grief. Fill my eyes with healing tears of rage.

I change my inner perception and the outer reveals the beauty so long obscured by my own attitude. I concentrate on my inner vision and find my outer view transformed.
— Daily Word

When we see something familiar like an old chair or a tree as if for the first time and we feel its incredible beauty, we know that somehow our inner perception has changed and we have been allowed a peek at the truth.

If only we could always see clearly. Most of the time our vision is impaired. We miss the magic and everything looks dull. Usually what clouds our seeing is judgment. Before we ever look we've made a judgment. It covers our eyes and allows us to see only what it wants us to see.

Prayer and meditation help clear away the judgments that cover our eyes. So do quiet moments of reflection, spiritual reading, journal work, walks in nature. Our inner perception changes and the outer world looks more friendly, more beautiful. Truth reappears and we love what we see, including ourselves.

I will look at myself today as if for the first time. I will pray for the vision to see clearly how beautiful I am.

You are the best friend you will ever have.
In the presence of your true self you will
become the most peaceful, the most
relaxed, the most natural person possible.
— *Bartholomew*

Our endless search for The Right Person keeps
many of us unnecessarily busy. We're always
looking for that person who will cure our loneliness,
make us feel good about ourselves, and make us
feel whole.

Yet wholeness and happiness aren't things other
people can give us. They're gifts we give ourselves.

All along the best friend and life partner we could
possibly want, we already have. In our search for
happiness from "out there," we may have neglected
and abandoned our relationship to our self. Like
any good friend, we deserve attention and respect.
The more we attend to our self, the happier we'll be.

I am the right person for me. I will enjoy my company
today. I will be a very attentive, loving friend to myself.

*Let there be beauty and strength, power
and compassion, honor and humility, mirth
and reverence within you.*

— Starhawk

Balance and harmony. It's easy to get out of balance and not notice. Weeks, months, or years can pass before we realize we haven't had any fun, or we've forgotten our goals, or we haven't been meditating, or maybe we've been eating mounds of ice cream every night.

If our imbalance manifested itself in an easy to understand way we'd probably walk around listing dramatically to one side like a sinking ship. Yet our bodies do tell us when we're out of balance. But they do it more subtly. Illness is a signal. It's one way our body tells us we're out of balance and harmony.

Illness, depression, or anxiety can be signals for us to take an honest inventory of ourselves. It's important for us to take time to check in and ask ourselves how we feel about the way we're living our lives. When we realize we've been out of balance, we can begin to rectify and restore balance.

I seek harmony and balance. I allow all parts of myself expression. I am happy, whole, and complete.

No one can ask another to be healed.
But he can let himself be healed, and
thus offer the other what he has received.
Who can bestow upon another what he
does not have? And who can share what
he denies himself?
— *A Course in Miracles*

Many of us are healers and helpers and lovers
of people with AIDS. Regardless of how we are
affected, AIDS can offer us a gift if we are open to
it. Like a searchlight, AIDS can shed light on places
in *our* lives where we have work to do too.

Maybe we need to learn to give without being attached to the outcome. Maybe we're too attached
to a career, relationship, or money. Maybe the AIDS
searchlight shines on our low self-esteem. Whatever
is exposed, now is the time to get help and accept
healing for ourselves.

And so we meditate — not just suggest it for
others. We take time to eat right, relax, and exercise. We learn to live in the present. We learn to
love ourselves unconditionally. Then, helping others
is easy. We just show up.

I help heal because I am being healed. I gratefully
accept loving energy, healing light, and divine love in
my life now.

April

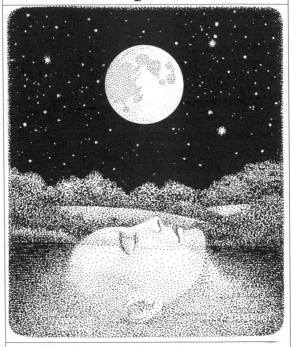

Today I flow with the river. I am one with the moon. I am peaceful and calm. I forgive myself and everyone else.

As long as we're taught to believe we are victims to whatever health hazards come our way we won't have the necessary strength to change the conditions that gave us the trouble in the first place.
— *Margo Adair*

No disease in modern history has captured attention as AIDS has. Much of the fear and hysteria comes from a belief that our only hope lies in medical science saving us with a "cure." And the medical world is failing us. AIDS is proving more powerful than science.

We need to recognize that our bodies do the healing. Our doctors and healers can help, but in the end, we do the healing. Our job is to create the best conditions for the healing to take place.

If, through the miracle of healing, our bodies can mend a broken leg, they can also mend a broken immune system. One miracle isn't harder to do than another. We need to expect, prepare for, and accept miracles in our lives. We are not helpless victims. We are powerful, magical, and miraculous.

I am a miracle of life. My body performs miracles of healing and mending. I am powerful, whole, and complete.

Your mind
cannot possibly understand God.
Your heart already knows.
Minds were designed for carrying out
the orders of the heart.
                                    — *Emmanuel*

Many of us have a hard time with the idea of a Higher Power or God because our rational mind doesn't make room for something we can't see or touch. Our mind tells us that what we see is what we get, nothing else. Yet, a life based only on what our rational mind tells us can be dry and unsatisfying.

The problem is: we let our mind lead our heart when we actually work best with our heart leading our mind.

With our heart leading us, we'll probably have no problem with Higher Power concepts. Heart doesn't bother with ideology or theology; it just connects to the source of all power and lets the energy flow.

I sit quietly, breathe deeply, and bring my awareness to my heart. Today I will follow the guidance of my heart.

*There is no other preparation for death
except opening to the present. If you are
here now, you'll be there then.*
— Stephen Levine

"How do I want to die?" is a hard question, a question most of us didn't think we'd be asking ourselves quite yet. Nevertheless, here we are, and it's a good question.

For most of us, the answer is probably simple. When we die, we want to be present, all our senses ready for whatever is going to happen next.

So it seems best to begin practicing right now. We can try to be present in each moment, all senses working in the now.

It takes practice. Many of us know how to go through life part dead, numbed by alcohol, other drugs, sugar, worry, fear. That's all we knew. But now we have a choice. We can choose to live fully present, crisply alive. We can choose to be living, not numb.

Please help me be present, fully alive, vibrant, and awake.

Man is composed of such elements as vital breath, deeds, thought, and the senses — all of them deriving their being from the Self. They have come out of the Self, and in the Self they ultimately disappear — even as the waters of a river disappear in the sea.

— IV Prasna, Upanishad

It's easy to become attached to our ego selves — the personalities that we develop over the years. We hang on to our negative behaviors, such as using alcohol and other drugs, because that's who we think we are. Without them, we're afraid we'll be dull and boring. But they have little to do with who we really are. They came from not knowing ourselves, not from knowing.

As we let go of our addictions, we became more interesting, not less. As negative behavior slips away, we begin to sparkle.

We begin a voyage of discovery, a search for our true selves and purpose. We learn the paradox: when we let go of what we thought made us unique, we discover how special we really are.

Today I will connect to my true self and become willing to let go of all behavior that keeps me from becoming that person.

Nor is it an objection to say that we must understand a prayer if it is to have its true effect. That simply is not the case. Who understands the wisdom of a flower? Yet we can take pleasure in it.
— *Rudolph Steiner*

Spiritual awakenings usually happen when we surrender our understanding. We give it up — all the intellectualism and efforts to figure it out. Usually, the big breakthroughs happen when we don't understand. We just hurt, and in this confusion, we end up praying.

Prayer comes in many forms. Sometimes it's just talking, being honest with whoever or whatever is listening in the world of spirit. Other times, prayer means repeating verses we memorize. For most of us, those are the prayers of our childhood. When we really need help the most, it doesn't matter what form we use or what prayer we say. It's our surrendering that counts.

Prayers and affirmations can work. We don't need to know why to take advantage of the results.

Today I will pray. I will humbly offer a simple prayer of my own, or I will repeat one that I remember.

Just as the moon only reflects its light in a pool, so the mind, empty and unattached, does not know itself and the outside world as two things.
— *The Gospel According to Zen*

We easily forget our unity and separate ourselves into an "us" camp and a "them" camp. We divide on all sorts of issues: gay/straight, diagnosis/non-diagnosis, black/white, male/female. Sometimes we divide on differences of principle, but often divisions result because we rehearse conflict, expect disagreement, look for the advantage, and compete to win.

There is an alternative. Instead of rehearsing conflict in our heads, we can open up to the possibility that we don't know the best solution. We can begin to see a different reality than "Us versus Them." We can begin to see that we are all one. We recognize unity and project love.

The experience of AIDS is teaching us how to be more loving within our groups and across group lines. We are learning new ways of being in community.

Today I flow with the river. I am one with the moon. I am peaceful and calm. I forgive myself and everyone else.

Listening with undivided attention and unconditional love is perhaps the greatest gift we can extend to others.
— Gerald Jampolsky

We don't often see how important we are to other people, but each of us makes a big difference. Listening, accepting, and paying attention may be the most important thing we can do for the people in our lives.

Many of us don't get listened to enough about how AIDS is affecting us. We think nobody wants to hear about it anymore, so we walk around numb with grief. But people are willing to listen, especially if they know that they will be listened to in return. These exchanges can allow us to cry, talk, rage, and be heard.

Listening is easier when we are willing to accept other people unconditionally and know we are not responsible for their feelings. We don't need to fix anybody or anything; we only need to listen.

I will listen and love today. I will give people the greatest gift I can — my attention. I will also make sure that I am listened to and loved. I will ask for what I need.

AIDS has been a transformative process for me. It's turned me from a person living in fear to a person who loves himself. I let others love me too. My walls are coming down.
— George Melton, person recovering from AIDS

And the walls come tumbling down. Or, at least they start to crumble. Whether they come down in a crash or little by little, the barriers we've placed around us begin to disappear as we learn to establish clear, reasonable boundaries.

Many of us grew up in homes where the adults who should have looked after us didn't. As a result, we often felt violated, afraid, and ashamed. We became adults who were afraid that if people got close they would hurt us, leave us, or both.

But we are not children anymore. We can provide the scared child inside us the protection he or she needs. And we are learning that people don't go away when they find out who we are. In fact, our humanness draws people to us.

Today I will comfort and protect the child inside me. I will love myself, and I will gratefully acknowledge the love coming to me from other people.

We must substitute faith for fear, for fear is only inverted faith; it is faith in evil instead of good.
— *Florence Scovel Shinn*

Fear is the big hurdle. Many of us spent most of our lives living in fear, sure that the world would treat us badly. And if we thought there was a God, we believed he was an old man just waiting to punish us or make us feel guilty. We rehearsed conflict, expected opposition, and were ready for the worst.

Now we are asked to have a faith. We are asked to believe that we are being cared for by a force of good. We are asked to let go of fear. At first this seems impossible. How can we make such a drastic change? Then we realize the only difference between faith and fear is that we expect good things instead of bad things.

Just the fact that we are reading this book means we have hope; we have a suspicion that there might be a better way of looking at the world. The real test is not whether faith makes more sense than fear. The real test is how our lives change. Is life better when we trust in a force for good?

Today I exchange fear for faith. I trust that my welfare is being looked after. I am safe and secure. I am blessed.

I went through a two-month period when I would take AZT from one hand and vodka from the other. One hand wanted to live. One hand wanted to die.
  — Mark Christopherson,
    person with AIDS

For many of us, to drink is to die. Using alcohol means we're wrecking our immune systems just when we need them most. With AIDS, drinking seems crazy, yet not drinking might seem crazy too. After all, what better reason to drink than AIDS? But then, many of us could always find a good reason to drink.

The point now is to find a good reason to be sober. And the reason is simple: we decide that we want to live. Every day that we are clean and sober we renew our affirmation for life. Whether or not we have a problem with alcohol or other drugs, we can all understand what it means to say, "Yes, I want to live." It is the heart of our relationship with ourselves. If we affirm this decision in our lives, we are more loving to ourselves and to the people around us.

I can be clean and sober today. Today I will say yes to life in everything I do.

Enlightened ones are very rarely holy.
— *Bartholomew*

Sometimes we think that being spiritual means living up to images that are impossible to copy, like Jesus and Buddha. What they were really like when they walked the earth, we don't really know. Nevertheless, we think we should try to be like them. So whenever we feel angry, resentful, jealous, afraid, or greedy, we try to quickly stamp out our feelings. After all, we think we should be further along the spiritual path and above those negative emotions.

But we're still human, and these emotions exist. Every time we try to disown one of our feelings we disown part of ourselves. When we deny them or ignore them we lose a part of ourselves that deserves to be loved unconditionally.

Whenever a feeling pops up that we'd rather deny than express, we can try accepting ourselves for having the feeling and accept the feeling too. We can imagine ourselves as enlightened beings who freely express a brilliant rainbow of feelings.

Today I will allow myself to feel any emotions that rise up. I will rejoice in my humanness.

Disease can be seen as a call for personal transformation through metamorphosis. It is a transition from death of your old self into the birth of your new.
— Tom O'Connor, person with ARC

When we get sick, it's easy to assume we did something to cause the illness. With AIDS, all we have to do is listen to the judgers and moralists. They're always telling us what we did wrong.

But it's best not to listen to them. Guilt and shame weaken our immunity and steal our energy.

And there is still no explanation why some people get sick and other people don't. Except that some of us may need the opportunity illness gives us to make changes.

We always have a choice. We can see disease as a terrible retribution for our sins. Or we can see whatever happens as another opportunity to make changes, transform, and become new people.

I now look at each new experience with wonder and curiosity. What does the universe have in store for me today? What can I learn? What can I change?

> *. . . a society can be judged according to the number and range of options of consequence it makes open to its people.*
> — *Norman Cousins*

The threat of dying young has forced many of us to look at our situations and reassess our goals. Are we seeing all the options the universe has to offer? Are we automatically closing doors because our belief systems say, "I can't do that, have that, be that"?

Many of us have believed that because we are gay, black, Hispanic, poor, or chemically dependent, we don't have options. We may have thought we have to take what the world hands out. So we buried our talents, packed away our dreams, and lost contact with our creative selves.

One way society keeps its doors closed is by convincing us we can't open them. Our first step is to open the doors of possibility in our minds. We must imagine, dream, and believe.

Today I courageously unlock all the doors of possibility in my mind. I am free to be and express all that I am.

Your attitude of mind is important. A faith-filled, loving, expectant attitude will speed up the healing processes of your body.
— *James E. Sweaney*

Truly, the results are in. Even the most pragmatic doctors will admit that a positive, hopeful attitude helps a person recover from illness.

When we expect to be up and about in a few days, we're more likely to be up and about in a few days. When we trust our healers and our Higher Power, we are able to relax and let our body repair itself.

When we surround ourselves with love and acceptance and breathe in its golden energy, we give even the most tired immune system extra power and possibility.

I am one body, mind, and spirit. I surround my entire self with golden white light. I breathe in its healing energy. I exhale all foreign bodies. I continue to breathe in golden healing light and exhale all debris until I am completely filled with the radiant energy of love.

*And to my surprise, instead of dying — I
was reborn. I knew to the core of my being
that I had healed myself. I was in a state
of grace, a place of total love and forgiveness. I was bounding with energy.*
— Tony Petzel, person with AIDS

The stories about healing are endless. It often
seems that AIDS is here to show us where we need
healing and to teach us how to heal. Whether we
have a diagnosis or not, we are finding places in
our lives that need nurturing, encouragement, and
kind attention.

AIDS is helping us transform. Sometimes this
is apparent in dramatic ways, other times it is
more subtle. For example, when we feel warm and
loving toward ourselves, when in the past we would
have been cold and critical, we know we have
been transformed.

Every time we are tolerant, we have been
transformed. Every moment we live fully in the
present, not worried about tomorrow or yesterday,
is a rebirth experience.

*Throughout this day, when my mind wanders, I will
bring myself back to the present. I will pay attention
to transformations taking place in my life.*

Burn bright flame within me
Symbol of eternal fire
Of the people we do be
And the people part of me
All One many parts
Single fire of flaming hearts.
— *Sacred Chant*

Where will our spirit go when we die? Where will our fire go? Where has the fire gone that lit up the eyes of our friends? When they died, what happened to it?

Are their lights extinguished, or are they part of the fire that we are all connected to, draw energy from, warm ourselves by, and take comfort in?

When people who we don't even know die, and we feel sad, is that because we are all connected?

And if we are very quiet, can we feel their loving energy near us, surrounding us, glowing, warming, protecting, friendly, loving light energy?

I am connected to the one source of all light. So are my friends. I feel their peaceful presence and trust they feel mine.

It is wonderful to move from happiness to depression, when you are moving! It is when you are not moving that you become afraid and take that fear into your body, which becomes rigid, stiff, and constricted!
— Mary Margaret Moore

If we were truly spiritual, we would be happy, peaceful, and content all the time. Right? Wrong.

While others may not always understand our bad moods, being angry and saddened may be exactly where we need to be. If that's how we feel, the worst thing we can do is deny it. Denying our feelings is like cutting off an important part of ourselves because we think it isn't acceptable.

When we accept all our feelings, they keep moving and we become able to experience a full range of emotions. We become more aware of how vast we are. When we accept our feelings, all of them, then we love ourselves.

I love moving from one emotion to another. I love and appreciate the full rainbow of my emotions.

In the face of uncertainty there is nothing wrong with hope.
   — *Carl and Stephanie Simonton*

All life is uncertain. Why should we now decide that having AIDS is a hopeless predicament? That's ridiculous.

So we hope. We expect a good outcome. We visualize a happy result. We say, "I hope for this and I can see it happening."

Hope is present and powerful. Hope is faith in movement and change, and comes from a secure knowledge that we are in the care of a Power larger than ourselves. Hope is creative. Hope is the simple knowledge that miracles happen every day. They are the natural result of hope. They are only unusual or unexplainable to people who are afraid to hope.

Hope is honest and never false.

I am grateful for the miracles happening today in my life. I am grateful for the love and peace that hope gives me.

I'm powerless over other people's dying.
— David Grundy

Many of us have spent years confused about where we are powerful and where we are powerless. We thought we were powerful over alcohol, other drugs, and other people. On the other hand, we also believed we were powerless over how we reacted to people and events. If we exploded in anger, that was just the way we were and it couldn't be helped.

The truth is, many of us are absolutely powerless over alcohol and other drugs. But we are powerful over our reactions to people and events. Our attitude determines our reactions, and we do have the power to change our attitudes.

And finally, we're powerless over other people. We can try to get people to work their program the way we want them to. We can try to keep someone from dying. Ultimately, though we have no control over other people living and dying. When we accept this, life is easier for us and for the people around us.

Help me let go of other people's living and dying. Help me focus on my life and my attitude. Help me to always remember that all I have to give is love.

*[Compassion] means, as far as I under-
stand it, the ability to see how it all is. As
long as you have certain desires about how
it ought to be you can't see how it is.*
— *Ram Dass*

AIDS is teaching us compassion. We're learning
there is no right or wrong way to have AIDS or love
a person with AIDS.

We're learning that the most important thing we
can do is listen with an open mind and an open
heart, trying to understand how things are for
another person.

If we can be compassionate with others, we can
also be compassionate with ourselves. Just as we
accept others, we need to accept ourselves, without
judgment, blame, or guilt. In fact, if we want to be
compassionate to others, the place to begin is at
home. As we accept ourselves, unconditionally, we
find it easier to do the same for others.

*I let go of all judgments about myself, about other
people, and about how life ought to be. I listen to myself
and others with an open heart.*

Macrobiotics is based on the idea that you
are the master of yourself — not bacteria,
doctors, scientists, ministers, philosophers
or dietitians — not even macrobiotic ones.
— *Herman Aihara*

AIDS is teaching many of us about diet. We're talking to nutritionists; we're cutting out additives, chemicals, sugar. We're a lot more careful about what we put into our bodies.

We're learning about moderation and balance and the joy they can bring. For many of us, this is a revelation. We once wanted more, more, more. Now, we're learning that the empty, aching hole inside us needs to be filled with love.

Now, we understand that more chemicals, a higher high, or sex won't fill that emptiness. We are replacing our fear with love and learning that our bodies have limits. We cannot keep doing bad things to our bodies without bad results. By accepting ourselves and living within those limits, we demonstrate self-love.

I joyously accept my limits. I am happy and free. I listen to others and take counsel with myself. I love the choices I make today.

Everyday ask yourself the question, "Do I want to experience Peace of Mind or do I want to experience Conflict?"
— *Gerald Jampolsky*

This question reminds us that we always have a choice. We can follow the path of conflict or the path of peace.

The point is to remember we are choosing, not simply reacting. In the morning and all through the day, when we are anxious or afraid, we can step out of our anxiety and choose peace.

The problem is, we often forget we have a choice. We stay in conflict and wear out our body and soul. The more worried and fearful we become, the harder it is to remember that we have a way out.

That's why some daily routines help. When praying, meditating, or writing in our journal, in these moments of reflection and quiet, we remember we have choices. We can choose to love; we can choose peace of mind.

I am grateful for the quiet time I take. Help me to always remember that I have the power to choose.

Refusal to hope is nothing more than a decision to die. I know there are people alive today because I gave them hope and told them they didn't have to die.
— Bernie Siegel

A lot of doctors are afraid of giving what they call "false hope." Many AIDS caregivers learn about false hope from their doctors and are afraid they might spread it too.

But how can hope be false? Hope is hope. It is always true. Hope is real.

Life force is an amazing energy. While it runs through our bodies, it is capable of anything. No one can limit our life force; through it we connect to the rest of the universe.

As long as the force of life runs through us there is always hope. It means we are still connected and open to being flooded with healing light and love.

I give and receive the gift of hope. I believe in the creative power of my life. I am connected to all power, all light, all love.

All of life is maintenance. Taking care of
things. That's the pleasant part.
— Armistead Maupin

Many of us have been addicted to excitement.
Each night out had to compete with the best and
most exciting night we'd ever had. We were driven
and compulsive. We neglected our bodies, environment, relationships, and emotional needs. The
excitement we furiously searched for never really
satisfied us, so we kept looking for more.

That was then. Now we can commit to a new
way of living. We can commit to enjoying the thrill
of taking good care of ourselves. When we bring
our minds to the present moment and pay loving
attention to ourselves, each mundane routine can
become a healing ritual.

When the mind and body are united (when
we're thinking about what we're doing), even
housecleaning can bring serenity. We begin to
realize that showing self-love in daily actions is
deeply satisfying.

When I take good care of myself I say, "I love you"
loud and clear. Today I will make my daily chores
rituals of love and healing.

I prayed, "Please don't let me die without knowing what this is about. If I die that's okay, I don't care, but just let me learn what this is about." From that point on, things began to change. I quit searching for a physical healing. It was a spiritual healing. My spirit was sick and my body just reflected that.

— George Melton, person recovering from AIDS

There is a big difference between "What did I do to deserve this?" and "What can I learn from this?" One attitude sticks us with guilt. The other frees us from judgment and blame.

AIDS is not punishment; it is not a symbol of failure. AIDS may be a symbol of a neglected or wounded spirit. Which means we also need to attend to our emotional and spiritual recovery.

Our treatment might include: walking in the woods or park, talking with people who love and support us in our spiritual healing (people also on a spiritual path), reading, praying, and searching out guides and teachers, and being as kind and loving to ourselves as we can be, one day at a time.

I am at work healing my Spirit. When I feel pain, I bring it into my heart, surround it in love, and let it go.

You are cradled in the infinite love of God, and yet, you must open your heart to your own humanness completely and totally for that love to heal you.

— *Emmanuel*

We know what it feels like to open our hearts to others. We can accept their humanness. It's harder to accept our own. That means accepting our mistakes, our imperfections, our mediocrity. It means being a peer, equal to others, just one person in a circle — neither better than, nor less than others.

When we open our hearts to our humanness, we accept our quirks, the things that make us unique and endear us to others. We also acknowledge, accept, and honor our needs. Nothing stamps us as human more clearly than needing help from other people. We all need love, caring, affection. We need to be listened to, held, touched, appreciated. We need help solving our problems. We need others.

I open my heart to my humanness. I accept my needs, my desires, my wants, my problems, my personality, and my limitations. What a relief to relax and just be a human being.

Healing is to be found only when, having found God in ourselves, we pour out unselfishly into the world in thought, feelings and actions what we have won.
— *Rudolph Steiner*

Many of us know that the quality of our sober lives improves dramatically when we carry the message of recovery to other people. It helps us gain a measure of peace, and we want those who still suffer to have what we have.

The big secret we have to tell is this: I'm a good person; I deserve help. You're a good person; you deserve help. We don't have to do this alone.

The minute we turn to helping someone, our wounds begin to heal. We give a little and receive a lot. We see our pain reflected in the eyes of others, and through our compassion for them, they heal us.

So it is with AIDS. We find strength when we work together to dissolve the blocks to healing and trace the roots of our fear. Giving hope, we receive hope.

I am grateful for an awakened spirit. I bless those who gave me a chance to share what I have found. They are my healers.

I will seek the lost, and I will bring back the strayed, and I will bind up the crippled, and I will strengthen the weak, and the fat and strong I will watch over, I will feed them in justice.

— Ezekiel 34:16

How easy to lose faith in the laws of the universe, to see only pain and despair. How easy to act and think like a victim.

But all of us have been promised healing. Every illness comes with the promise of healing. Every question has the promise of an answer.

When we turn for help, we remember the balance, the prayer and the answer to prayer. Out of our isolation and loneliness we turn to a Higher Power, to our friends, to people in the program, to our support system, and we are promised understanding and relief.

Our sanity returns. We come to believe in and rely on a Power greater than ourselves. We trust the promise and our spirit begins to heal.

I trust that when I pray, I am heard, I am looked after, I am in divine safety.

Day after day the sun rises in the east;
Day after day the sun sets in the west.
— The Gospel According to Zen

"Don't take yourself too seriously" is a little warning we sometimes need. Too often we grit our teeth, put on a serious face, and trudge off to do battle with the world. After all, AIDS is very serious business.

Before we know it, our sense of humor is out the window. People annoy us. Little irritations build up. Days slip away and we forget to do the things that give us pleasure. We forget to have fun. We're busy preparing for tomorrow and not living today; we forget that all we really can live is today. All that really counts is how we live today.

So let's not take ourselves too seriously. Let's remember to poke fun at ourselves and have fun. Let's remember to pay attention to the world around us. As we do, we can take a deep breath, sigh, and remember that living with AIDS is more manageable one day at a time.

Today I will laugh and enjoy myself. I will live as much as I can, as good as I can, today.

*Peace be to you to whom is healing offered.
And you will learn that peace is given you
when you accept the healing for yourself.*
— *A Course in Miracles*

For many of us affected by AIDS, it's easier to be understanding than it is to be understood. It's easier to listen than to be heard. It's easier to hold someone in our arms than it is to be held. But we are asked to do just that. We are asked to accept love for ourselves and let others care for us.

What relief we experience when we realize that we, too, get to be just one person in a circle of people. What a revelation! The love, caring, and fellowship that we wish for others is extended to us. We get to share our feelings and let others listen sympathetically. We get to be heard and to listen without having to know any answers. In fact, the most important thing we can do is accept the love that is being given to us by our friends, our support groups, and our Higher Power.

Today I will relax deeply. When I attend meetings and support groups I will let the love of the group cleanse me, envelop me, and heal me.

May

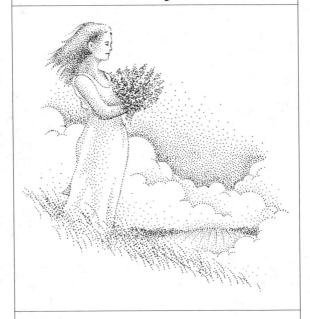

I imagine myself walking in a heavenly garden where I joyfully pick flowers that brighten my soul. The flowers are my teachers, books, and guides. The bouquet I make is my own unique spiritual practice.

I really believe we have the ability to heal ourselves and that we are here to teach the planet about love.
— *Gregory, person with AIDS*

We have the ability to heal ourselves. Our healing happens when we recognize our connection to each other and to the earth. Much of our lives we believed in a system of me and I. It didn't work very well. Now, as we begin living a belief system based on *us* and *we*, we find unlimited power. Impossible tasks are now possible — like not drinking; or using drugs or smoking.

Now, rather than seeing the world as a hostile place to live, we are becoming conscious of our unity with all living things. Just as alcoholism and addiction to other drugs might have taught us before, now AIDS is teaching us the amazing paradox: only when we admit our weakness and our need for help do we gain the power to accomplish the impossible.

None of us can fight AIDS alone. By coming together for healing, we are learning big lessons about power and strength. We are learning that it is our true nature to be loving and supportive.

Today I will tap deep into the earth and connect to the breathing, living Mother of us all. I will ask Her to heal us.

To love oneself is the beginning of a life-long romance.

— Oscar Wilde

If I were in the midst of the most perfect, wonderful love affair, what would my lover do for me? What would I do for my lover?

If we feel embarrassed or self-conscious by these questions, we may believe that we don't deserve to be happily, gloriously in love. When these old beliefs pop up we can just throw them out the window. We do deserve and we can have a magical life. It begins when we start loving ourselves — in practice, not just in theory.

So, how do we demonstrate our self-love? Do we say, "I love you" regularly, often, every chance we get? Do we give ourselves little gifts? Do we smile at ourselves and hug ourselves and compliment ourselves? Do we give ourselves enough rest and exercise and time for meditation? Do we do all those things that say, "You deserve perfect health and happiness"?

Today I will live as though I'm in a wild, glorious, never-ending love affair with myself. I will not be embarrassed or shy about demonstrating my self-love. I will do at least one thing that's a little outrageous or a little corny that says, I love you.

So many people have come to feel that illness is inevitable and that all must die of something, that the energy field emanated by these attitudes is actually attracting illness through acceptance of it as inevitable. Health is actually the way....

— *Right Use of Will*

There's a lot of energy invested in AIDS as a way to die. Many of us feel as if the circle is closing in on us as one by one our friends and acquaintances are diagnosed with AIDS or ARC. It's hard not to end up with a tremendous fear of AIDS and an attitude that it's inevitable.

We have a choice. We can go along with the prevailing fear, or we can decide that illness is not inevitable and then do what we can to attract energy, vitality, and health. We can focus on our spiritual journey and affirm our progress toward living fuller lives. We can ask those around us to join us in that direction. We can surround ourselves with positive people and protective white light.

I let go of all belief systems that attract illness. Today I will imagine the world filled with people who are also radiating powerful, positive healing energy.

Grandmother Earth hear me! The two-leggeds, the four-leggeds, the wingeds, and all that moves upon You are Your children. With all beings and all things we shall be as relatives; just as we are related to you O Mother.

— *Black Elk*

When we begin to recognize our relatedness to birds, animals, trees, other people, we step out of the illusion of separateness and we begin to heal our spirit.

But addiction can keep us stuck in the despair of being alone and unloveable. Whatever our addiction, our core belief is the same: we believe we're not good enough and that if people find out who we are they'll leave.

Recovery brings us into community with people who don't leave or judge us when we disclose the truth about who we are. We learn we are not alone. Other people share our feelings and no one is shocked at how "bad" we've been.

We begin to believe that we too are children of the universe. We are related and equal to all living things. We are loved unconditionally.

I will honor my Mother, the Earth, and all living things. I will be clean and sober today.

*This moment is the only moment there is,
and it is for love. In this moment there is
no guilt or fear.*
— Gerald Jampolsky

In the spring, when lilacs bloom, it's easy to believe that this moment is for love. In the spring, when the earth is reborn, when dandelions are everywhere, and birds build nests, and the ground is warm, and our bodies relax, and we sit in the sun and sigh, we let winter's tension melt away and remember once again what it feels like to let go.

Our faith returns in the spring. We feel our connection to all living things. In the spring, it's easier to notice the breeze and the green and the blue. And when we notice, we live in the moment. When we notice, we can believe with our mind and body that the world is for love.

If because of AIDS, we pay attention to spring more this year, if we notice more, then AIDS carries a gift. If because of AIDS, we live more in the moment, knowing that this is the only moment there is, then AIDS carries a gift. If this spring we can sigh and let go and remember that love is all, there is no guilt or fear, then we are home.

This moment is the only moment there is, and it is for love.

Heal a symptom by asking what it has to tell you. Every time you suppress a symptom you're saying to your body, "I don't love you. I don't love your messages."
— *George Melton, person recovering from AIDS*

When we ignore symptoms, we ignore our body's messages. How else does our body get our attention?

AIDS may be a symptom. Certainly opportunistic infections such as cancer, pneumonia, shingles, and thrush are symptoms. We can ask our throat, our tongue, or skin, lungs, or brain, "What do you have to tell me? I love you and I appreciate your message. Help me to understand. You have my full attention."

Then, if we sit or lie still and listen, with our minds focused on that body part we are trying to understand, we'll get an answer. We may want to try placing our left hand on our symptom and our right hand on our heart. Once we begin to listen, we make room for understanding. And we give our symptoms the chance to move out.

Until we correct what needs correcting, we may find it hard to get rid of our symptoms.

I listen to and trust my body. I listen respectfully to my symptoms and lovingly release them.

> *As I said before, it's that blazing determination that is necessary. And the end of helplessness is the beginning, it seems to me, of health.*
>
> — *Norman Cousins*

If we grew up accustomed to turning our power over to other people (parents, teachers, or other authority figures), an AIDS diagnosis or a positive HIV test can mean we once again give our power away, this time to our doctors. On the other hand, this could be the perfect chance to stop giving away our power and take responsibility for our recovery.

Taking full responsibility is exciting. It means that we decide that we aren't helpless, that there are lots of things we can do and it's up to us to choose the best alternatives for our health.

Once we take responsibility for what we do, we can let go of the outcome. Responsibility for outcomes we can turn over to a Higher Power, which is a big relief for our doctors, they don't have to be God any more, and neither do we.

I blaze with the fire of determination. I take responsibility for my life. I am glad to be alive.

For now we see in a mirror dimly, but then face to face. Now I know in part; then I shall understand fully, even as I have been fully understood.
— *I Corinthians 13:12*

Though we try to understand, we try to see clearly, most of the time it feels like we're walking through life in a fog. Even though we read books, go to meetings, talk to people, meditate, attend to our spiritual self as well as our physical self, most of the time, we're still in a fog.

We need to remind ourselves that all we have to do is live today and accept ourselves exactly as we are, even if we are foggy and confused.

We also need to trust that our Higher Power is clear, and that there is a place inside of us where there is clarity. So, when our vision is darkened and dim, we need to turn our eyes toward that light. There we find understanding and eternal knowing.

Please help me lift the fog of my misunderstanding. Help me always remember who I am. Help me turn my searching inward so that I may always live in the light.

The real voyage of discovery consists not in seeking new landscapes but in having new eyes.

— *Marcel Proust*

Sometimes we think our problems stem from being stuck in the wrong city, climate, relationship, or job. With a different view, the world would look better. The problem is, where you go, there you are. We take our problems with us.

Sooner or later we realize many of our problems have more to do with us than with the world. We begin to take responsibility for our lives. We start to sort out the things we can change from the things we can't. And we learn that a changed attitude can brighten most any neighborhood, relationship, or job.

Our vision clears. Then, if we do make changes, we have more to bring to the people we meet because we have new eyes.

I take responsibility for my happiness. I take responsibility for my attitude. I choose to see a world filled with abundance and love.

*Your distress about life might mean you
have been living for the wrong reason, not
that you have no reason for living.*
— Tom O'Connor, person with ARC

Many of us didn't look very closely at our lives
until AIDS came along. All of a sudden, our lives
have become more important, our time more precious. So, we decide to do some self-examining.

Often, we don't like what we see. How we're living doesn't match our ideals. We may discover that
we're still trying to please our parents or get back
at them. Or we try to avoid failure by not trying
at all. We may discover that we still fight a feeling
of not belonging, of being different.

Now, AIDS gives us a chance to stop and listen
to our inner voice, that voice encouraging us to move
toward what's real. AIDS says, do it now. Be as true
to yourself as you can possibly be. Stop living for
your parents, or your lover, or your children. Stop
trying to do what you think others want you to do.

*I am an original. I have my own reason for being. I
love discovering my true purpose, my true self. Every
moment of today I will try to be true to myself.*

Man spends his whole life running from feeling with the mistaken belief that you cannot bear the pain. But you have already borne the pain; what you have not done is to feel all that you are beyond that pain.
— *Bartholomew*

Many of us are afraid that our feelings will cause us pain. The truth is, running from them causes us pain. If we avoid our feelings, we learn what pain feels like, but we never find out what our feelings feel like.

If we stop running the pain stops. Of course, we are left with a whole lot of unexpressed feelings, feelings accumulated from many years of living in fear. This means we've got work to do. But we've also got a chance to finally live in the present and experience our feelings as they happen.

We begin to feel sadness, grief, anger, and joy. We begin to express all of our feelings. We cry, laugh, and scream. We release, expand, flow, and feel. We begin to move.

Help me start feeling and stop running. Release me from the constriction of anxiety and fear so that I may start to vibrate and move into total aliveness.

We planted flowers last year and I didn't know if I'd be alive to see them come up. Yesterday they were blooming. We decided to dig up more yard and plant more flowers.
— Neal McHugh, person with AIDS

Every moment has the potential for healing. To take advantage of that healing, we must be present. To appreciate the miracle of a blooming flower, we must be present. To allow the light in, we must open to the light.

We can realize this healing potential when we let go of our separateness and recognize our unity — with the flower, the sunset, and other people. It can happen during a snowfall, while walking in the woods on a summer day. It can even happen in our doctor's office when we stop being two people, one helpless and the other helper, and we see just one person healing.

None of us know what next year will bring, but we all can "act as if." The act of faith has the power to heal and transform. We can plant more flowers.

I will make room for flowers in my life today. I am One with everyone and everything.

Tell your mothers.
  — Betty Boulanger, mother of a person
     with AIDS

One of the saddest themes that runs through the AIDS drama is family rejection. Many of us avoid sharing our diagnosis or our health status, or our grief with our family because we're afraid of their reaction.

AIDS can be an opportunity for all of us, including our families. It offers us the opportunity to work through all the old stuff, all the anger, resentment, disappointment, and guilt. It gives us a chance to forgive ourselves and our parents. It gives us the chance to heal all our relationships.

Each of us gets to decide who to share our diagnosis with. Sharing it with our families may be worth it. Unhealed family relationships can be very stressful, healed family relationships can be very helpful.

Today I will look at all the relationships that need to be healed in my life, including my relationship with my family.

One's ships come in over a calm sea.
— *Florence Scovel Shinn*

How calm am I today? How calm this moment? Is peace of mind my only goal or am I attached to lots of outcomes today? Am I concerned about what other people are going to do, say, or think? Am I trying to control events and manipulate people into doing what I want? Am I dwelling on the past or worried about the future?

Am I filled with resistance? Can I accept any adverse condition and let go of all resistance to it? Instead of trying to beat my problems into submission, can I let them melt away?

Where's my focus today? Am I checking in on my feelings? Or have I forgotten about me and wound myself up in someone else's drama?

What's my perspective today? Do I remember that I am divine? Or do I forget and feel alone and threatened? Am I my work, my job, my body, my growth, my disease? Or, am I centered, eternal, part of creation, one with everyone?

I am calm, grounded, centered, and secure in God's love. I am peaceful, calm, and serene. I remember who I am.

Love is patient and kind; love is not jealous or boastful; it is not arrogant or rude. Love does not insist on its own way; it is not irritable or resentful; it does not rejoice in wrong but rejoices in the right. Love bears all things, believes all things, hopes all things, endures all things.
— I Corinthians 13: 4-7

Many of our backgrounds fostered the idea that God was fearful, often angry and vengeful. Even if we don't believe in God now, we may still carry around that old idea — fear of a force that is waiting to trip us up.

Now, as adults, we have the option of developing our own idea of God or a Higher Power. And each of us may have a slightly different version. Usually, though, we choose to believe the God, or Nature, or the Great Spirit, or the Goddess is patient and kind, loving and caring.

As our concept of God changes we learn to relax, to let down our guard and trust. When we believe God accepts us, we accept ourselves. We become patient and kind and the world looks friendly, peaceful, and supportive.

I touch the source of love when I touch my heart. God is love and so am I.

Inner silence is where you will find yourself.
— *Mary Margaret Moore*

We can all talk about our jobs, families, and relationships. We can even talk about our behaviors — outrageous, odd, destructive, sad, silly, whatever. But when it comes to talking about who we really are, we may have a hard time keeping the conversation going. Who am I? What am I like? Our minds go blank.

For many of us, only when we stepped out of the haze of alcohol and other drugs or stepped into the safety of a support group, did we begin to discover who we were, separate from our behaviors.

At first, we could only see our reflections in the eyes of other people. We saw that other people liked us and saw in us something of value. Maybe they'd say something nice about us and we'd think, well, maybe I am like that.

The next stage of self-discovery happens in silence and solitude: hearing, accepting, feeling, listening, being.

Today I will become more acquainted with myself. I will sit in silence and listen.

If you feel like you're helping too much, stop it immediately.
— *Sondra Smalley*

AIDS gives us a wonderful opportunity to help others. There's so much to do — people to visit, children to care for, meals to prepare, organizations to run, funds to raise.

If we tend to be caretakers, AIDS can set us up to lose ourselves in the lives of others. But if we aren't taking good care of our own needs, resentments will start popping up. We may become irritable, controlling, and angry. We may think people aren't appreciative, and they're not doing what we want them to do. Our serenity is out the window, and our service becomes sharp and brittle instead of strong, flexible, and loving.

When we start to feel like we're doing too much, we need to stop. No matter what. The world will keep going without our effort. In the meantime, we need to take care of ourselves. We need to make sure our physical, emotional, and spiritual needs are being met.

I am a loving, creative helper because I take very good care of myself.

Put aside the need to know some future design and simply leave your life open to what is needed of it by the Divine forces.
— Emmanuel

AIDS makes us want to know what's going to happen, even more than we did before. Will we die? Will our friends die? Will we get sick? Will we recover?

In the meantime, between now and what's going to happen, there is the present. Today. Today we can let go of our need to know (and desire to control) and see if there are ways to be helpful instead. We can leave destiny up to destiny, to God or fate.

When we let go of the future, open to the present and make ourselves available to serve and extend love, we also open to miracles and magic. They only happen in the present.

If we are open to doing what is needed, we won't care about tomorrow. Whatever happens, we'll be fine. We don't need to worry about the future; we've got a job to do, love to extend, now. We're specially made to do just that.

Today I pray, thy will be done. Amen.

Do not take life's experiences too seriously. For in reality they are nothing but dream experiences. Play your part in life, but never forget that it is only a role.
— *Paramahansa Yogananda*

How easy to be so very serious. Life is often hard, and now there's AIDS, which we all know is very serious. So we put on a sober face and concentrate on beating the odds.

Before we know it we're not having any fun. We've lost our sense of humor. We forget to enjoy life. We forget that there are no real winners or losers. There's just living.

So, if we've been taking ourselves too seriously, we need to go looking for our sense of humor. Then we need to do something corny, silly, foolish, ridiculous, and out of character — anything, as long as it isn't serious.

Today I will ask the little child inside of me what he or she wants to do to have fun. I will check in many times today to make sure he or she is laughing, smiling, and happy.

Your problem is you're afraid to ac-
knowledge your own beauty. You're too
busy holding onto your unworthiness.
— *Ram Dass*

Today I will admit, accept, and acknowledge my beauty. All day long, I will take every chance I can to look into a mirror and say to myself, "You're beautiful. Your life is as it should be."

I will also be very attentive to any thoughts that seem to imply unworthiness. I will notice them and let them pass out of my head like fast-moving clouds across a summer sky. If they are persistent, I will ask myself why I am attached to ideas of unworthiness. Where do they come from and who would I hurt if I decided not to keep them anymore?

Today I am replacing those old thoughts with the truth that I am worthy; I am a beautiful child of the universe and deserve all good things. Today I lose all attachment to ideas of unworthiness. Today I focus on new and wonderful blessings already on their way.

Today it is easy to look in the mirror and say, "You're beautiful. I love you."

I am a beautiful child of the universe. Negative thoughts now drift away. They are replaced by a shining aware-ness of my own brilliance.

*A door opens wide when danger and
death approach. Somehow when we no
longer feel in control, we become available to deeper aliveness.*
— Richard Moss

The door opens and we walk through. We give
up. We let go. The illusion of control vanishes,
and we're standing naked and vulnerable. In
that moment we are aware that we are alive and
very human.

For many of us, that is what the beginning of recovery from alcohol and drug addiction was like.
We gave up and turned ourselves in. When we did,
we realized surrendering made us free.

AIDS is like that. It gives us the opportunity to
surrender to a deeper sense of aliveness. Vulnerable and afraid, we let go and trust our lives to a
Higher Power.

Now when life is scary, we don't have to run away.
We know that it's okay to be vulnerable. We know
that we are not alone and that we can risk letting go.

---

*I turn my control over and let go. I am alive and human
and vulnerable and surrounded by love.*

There is no right or wrong way to have this disease. Nor is there a right or wrong way for those without Aids to respond to their friends who have been diagnosed.
— *Keith Gann, person with AIDS*

What do you say when a friend tells you he or she has AIDS? What do you say to your father or mother, your son or daughter? And how do you tell your friends and family about your diagnosis?

Many of us have felt the discomfort of not knowing what to say or how to behave. All we need to remember is that we don't have to be the perfect person with AIDS or the perfect support person. We can just be present with another person and extend our love. Not perfectly. Not every time. Just as best we can. That's all we're called on to do.

Can we be accepting parents, lovers, family, and friends? Can we accept our family, lover, friends? All we're asked to do is be willing to move in the direction of loving acceptance. Not perfectly. Not every time. Just the best we can. Today.

I see a world of "we" today. Not a world of "us and them" or "they and me." I see people who love me just the way I am, just the best they can.

You can promote your healing by your thinking.

— *James E. Sweaney*

All the things we do to treat our illnesses can be helped along enormously by combining them with positive thoughts. For example, when we take vitamins we can say, "I'm thankful for the good effect these have on my health."

Positive affirmation and positive, life-enhancing visualizations will help whatever we do, whether we're taking chemotherapy, radiation, herbs, or acupuncture.

Cancer patients visualize their T-cells and macrophages gobbling up the cancer cells. People with Kaposi Sarcoma lesions imagine them disappearing. How we use our ability to image and visualize is limited only by our imaginations.

Affirmations such as, "My immune system is vibrant and powerful. I am filled with loving energy," tell us our healing is happening and progressing.

Today I will combine positive acting with positive thinking. I will be creative and imaginative and write positive notes to myself. My thoughts take an active role in my healing.

*Be not content with future happiness. It has
no meaning, and is not your just reward.
For you have cause for freedom now.*
— *A Course in Miracles*

Live a day at a time. Be here now. Live in the
present. Again and again we hear how important
it is to live in the moment, to focus on today. We
nod our heads in agreement as our minds drift off
to yesterday or tomorrow.

After all, we've been taught to worry about the
future: "Get good grades so you'll get a good job
or get into college.... Save money.... Plan
ahead." The motto is: Sacrifice now, be happy later.

Behind that thinking is a belief that we don't
deserve a wonderful life. We're taught to believe that
only after we've paid lots of dues and made ourselves nearly perfect, do we deserve happiness.
Wrong. We deserve happiness now. Life is happening now. Now is the only time anything ever
happens. This is it. This is real. We can have
wonderful lives now.

---

*I choose happiness now. I will pay attention to my
thoughts and actions and make sure I am not postponing my life, or putting off my feelings, or waiting
to be happy.*

> *. . . we ought never to minimize or underestimate the nature of the problems that confront us . . . we ought never to minimize or underestimate our ability to deal with them.*
>
> — *Norman Cousins*

Whether we like it or not, AIDS is here, and it's serious. There's no sense underestimating or denying AIDS. But the only alternative many of us see to denial is despair. So we bounce back and forth.

We achieve balance and harmony in the face of AIDS when we accept the seriousness of it and also remember who we are. We are children of God, capable of great power, capable of being filled with loving energy.

We can find that point of harmony and balance inside ourselves. It's where we connect with the power of the earth below and to the mystery of the sky above. We find it when we sit quietly, focus inward, and breathe. Then we know that we are not hopeless, helpless victims. Then we find the strength to deal with all life's challenges, including AIDS.

I am connected to the power of the universe. I breathe in love and light and exhale fear and darkness. I am confident and powerful. I am at peace.

A lot of drug addicts think AIDS is their punishment for being an addict.

— Kevin

There's a lot of guilt energy floating around in the world. Like a magnet, we can attract guilt and shame and other bad feelings to us.

There is an alternative. We can choose to let guilt and shame float by. We can let go of old ideas about God and punishment. Instead, we can be magnets for self-love, self-acceptance, and forgiveness. There's more than enough love, acceptance, and forgiveness floating around to satisfy each of us. And magically, the more we attract it and hold it in our hearts, the more there is for others.

It's a matter of choice. We can consciously choose love instead of fear, forgiveness instead of guilt. What a nice habit to get into — always moving toward the love.

I love myself exactly the way I am. I accept my addicted self. I accept my AIDS self. I accept my guilty self. I forgive myself.

> *. . . pray for one another that you may be
> healed. The prayer of a righteous man has
> great power in its effects.*
> — James 5:16

"I'll pray for you" can sound embarrassingly
old-fashioned and religious. Yet, we can pray for
each other. We can send our love through the air.
We can put our attention on our friends' well-being
and healing. We can think about people we know
in such a way as to place ourselves in connection, communication, and communion with them.
When we do, we establish intimacy. What could
be more intimate than holding someone in
your heart?

The wonderful thing about prayer is we don't
need to know it works before we do it. We can just
try. And though we may never know what effects
our prayer has on others, we can at least know our
prayers for others return to us as healing energy.

---

*I will try to be prayerful in all my thoughts today. I
will send prayers of healing and love to my friends and
people I know. I am grateful for this opportunity to be
anonymously helpful.*

Don't listen to negative people, negative doctors, or the media.
— *Tony Petzel, person with AIDS*

People are beginning to discover that AIDS is not a 100 percent fatal disease. Many of those who were sure it was aren't sure anymore. Some doctors once overly concerned about giving "false hope" are now hopeful. This is reason enough to stop listening to anyone who tells us that AIDS will kill us.

Most long-term AIDS survivors agree that it's best to stay clear of negative people, whether they're our neighbors, doctors, clergy persons, or friends.

We can choose who we spend time with, who we listen to, and what we believe. We get to have our own opinion and live by it. We always have a choice. Those who would limit us are only projecting their fear. We can bless them and let them go.

I listen to the sound of hope. I freely choose the path that's right for me.

Once you begin to believe there is help "out there," you will know it to be true.
— *Bartholomew*

Belief is a very misty concept. How do I know that I really believe? How do I know that my belief is genuine? If doubt creeps in does that cancel my belief? How much belief do I need?

The wonderful thing about belief is that it takes just a very little bit. A mere movement in the direction of believing is all we need. We don't need never-doubt-for-a-minute belief. We don't have to have a Rock-of-Ages unshakable faith. We only need a hunch, a suspicion that there might be a helping force in the world, a power beyond our ego and will.

All we need is a little willingness and a little open mindedness. And if we can't be willing, we can at least be willing to be willing, or willing to be willing to be willing.

That's all it takes. Once we open the door a crack it swings wide open on its own.

I am open to receiving help from powers I don't understand and forces I can't see.

The big first step is saying, "I can do something."
— *Tom O'Connor, person with ARC*

"I can do something." What a glorious, revolutionary statement. I am not a helpless AIDS victim. I am not at the mercy of AIDS survival statistics or a doctor's life expectancy predictions. The life force runs through me now. Nothing is more powerful. And I can do something.

I can call someone. I can go to a support group. I can go to a meeting. I can read a book about my immune system. I can eat a good meal. I can stay sober today. I can take a walk. I can meditate. I can pray. I can focus on my breathing. I can cry or laugh or scream or break a plate. I can ask for help. I can be willing to let miracles happen in my life.

I can focus my mind and heart in the right direction. And every move I make toward healing empowers me and makes me stronger.

I am an actor in my life. I take responsibility for my actions. I turn outcomes over to a Higher Power.

Buddha said the same thing about the good ox driver. The driver knows how much load the ox can carry, and he keeps the ox from being overloaded. You know your way and your state of mind. Do not carry too much.
— *Zen Mind, Beginner's Mind*

We push and push until we're at the edge and overwhelmed. We're overcommitted. There are too many meetings, hospital visits, appointments, too much work. We're moving too fast and not admitting it. It takes getting honest to admit that we need to slow down and relax. It takes willingness to let that happen.

It also takes courage. We need courage to say no to new commitments. We need courage to give ourselves more time to rest. Sometimes, those of us with AIDS need special doses of courage to admit and accept our changing limitations.

No matter how important our tasks, our first responsibility is to ourselves. We need to honor and respect our emotional and physical limits.

In other words, what Buddha was saying was, "Easy Does It."

I love and accept myself just the way I am. I honor and respect my limits. I am in tune to the rhythm of my life.

June

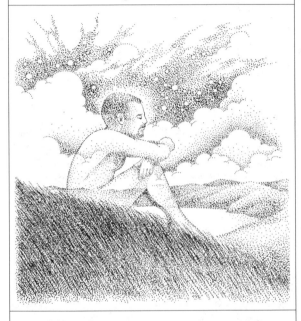

I sit quietly and allow my thoughts to pass. I imagine that I am a calm lake. I allow disturbing thoughts to drift away like clouds across the sky. I allow comfort and peace to surround and penetrate my body.

Let the beauty we love be what we do.
There are hundreds of ways to kneel and
kiss the ground.

— *Rumi, a Sufi poet*

Television, movies, and advertising tell us how we ought to be, what we should look like, how much money we should make, what we should do. They try to limit us by saying, "Only this kind of life is acceptable."

In real life, though, the people who attract our attention and hold it are people good at being themselves. The way they live is honest; they're true to themselves. Watching them, we know they are limited only by their creativity, not by what other people tell them.

Each of us is able to be like that. We can shine with integrity and purposeful living. We can start by honoring ourselves, paying attention to what makes us feel good, strong, and right.

Supporting others in the way they do things — giving them room to live lives of purpose and integrity — also moves us forward. We celebrate our differences and cheer each other along the way.

I push against the walls of my imagination to see who I am. I honor my true self.

*I am not a statistic. I don't have to accept
anything that doesn't fit in my heart.*
— Robert Levithan

Statistics are useful to insurance companies, not
to real people. Statistics about AIDS have been used
to scare the wits out of us. And those of us who,
despite the numbers, are still very much alive are
dismissed and discounted by the numbers people.

We don't have to buy the predictions based on
statistics. We have every right to reject other people's predictions. We are our own authorities.

Daily inventories help make sure we don't let
someone else's statistic, or premonition of disaster,
or projection of fear, or prediction into our field
of consciousness. If we pay attention, we can edit
our ideas; this is mine, but this belongs to someone else, it doesn't fit with what I believe.

---

*I always know what's right for me. I quietly listen to
my heart. I easily let go of beliefs that don't fit and
fears that aren't mine.*

*I believe Aids is only one symptom of a
planetary illness. Earth herself has been
pushed to the edge of collapse.*
— Keith Gann, person with AIDS

We are learning a lot about the earth as a living
organism. We can see the earth healing herself from
the damage caused by pollution and environmental
insanity. Of course, if we continue to abuse the
earth, she may lose her ability to heal herself.

This is the way it is for us too. It may be difficult to heal our bodies and minds after years of
polluting ourselves with chemicals and negative
thinking, but we do have that ability.

The first step is to stop polluting ourselves. For
that, we may need help. We need the support of
other people, the help of a Power greater than
ourselves. Then every day we stay clean and sober,
every day we eat right and get enough rest and
exercise, we bring ourselves back into balance. And
we help the earth restore herself to balance too.

*I am one with my Mother the Earth. We are both
healing.*

> *I now do things not so much because of ARC but because I want to grow and realize my full self. How ironic it is that we often have to face death to learn about life.*
> — Tom O'Connor, person with ARC

AIDS has led many of us into making changes that we probably would have put off for years. We decided we wanted to live, so we began eliminating those things that were self-destructive such as alcohol, other drugs, cigarettes, and junk food.

Then we learned that our addictions and compulsive behavior kept us cut off from other people, from our spirituality, and from our feelings. We discovered how exciting it is to have feelings and feel alive instead of running from them into numbness and oblivion. We learned that the fear of hurt is often more painful than hurt itself.

Ironically, this experience is teaching us that life can be wonderful, that our lives can be full and rich, that we can become the people we were born to be.

I am willing to experience hurt. I no longer live in terror of phantom feelings. I accept my feelings and surround them with love.

I asked my doctor what he thought I could do. He said, "Nothing." But I decided there were lots of things I could do. I'm not going to sit around and wait to get sick.
— Stephen Fish, HIV positive

Our worries carry a lot of power. If we invest energy expecting to get sick, we'll probably get sick. If we believe there's nothing to be done except wait and worry, we'll end up spending all our time thinking about the future and miss the present which is too bad. The future isn't here yet; the present is.

When we live in the present, we become powerful actors. We see choices to make that can make life better for us right now. The more energy we put into living in the present, into life-affirming and immune-enhancing behaviors, the more healthy we become.

So, if the people around us believe there is nothing that can be done, we need to find people who will support us in positive action, people who are also determined to live in the present.

Stepping out of a victim role and walking into an active state of taking responsibility for life is a wonderful way to live.

I act. I gladly take responsibility for my health. I am radiantly healthy and alive.

If I can just love you because here we are,
then you are free to grow as you need to
grow, because none of it's going to change
my feeling of love.

— *Ram Dass*

Can we love without conditions, strings, or expectations? Can we love someone just because, here we are? Yes, we can.

And if we're not doing it perfectly now, we can decide that's where we want to go. When we allow ourselves to love others as they are, we live in peace. We live in a space with plenty of room for all of us to be and expand into who we are becoming.

The alternative is conflict. Conflict in our relationships may be caused by the expectations and conditions we've placed on others. Maybe we aren't giving them the room they need to be who they are.

Instead of conflict, we can choose peace. We can allow others the space they need to grow without fear of losing our affection and our love. We give an incredible gift when we choose peace; we give the gift of freedom. The people we love are free to change, and we are free to let them.

I love others unconditionally. I remove all strings and requirements that I may have attached to my affection. I love myself without conditions too.

*Some [people] measure only problems and
fail to measure themselves.*
— *Norman Cousins*

It's easy to see AIDS in general, and our personal
condition in particular, as giant, overwhelming
problems. When we view ourselves as victims,
everything looks big and threatening. Many of us
have learned to look at the world this way because
the people we counted on to protect us when we
were young often let us down. We learned early
on that the world wasn't a friendly or safe place.

But we no longer need to look at the world
through the big frightened eyes of a child. We're
adults now, able to surround ourselves with protection and care; we're able to connect to other
people and to the power of the universe.

So when we measure ourselves, we must measure
a vastness that includes all our possibilities and connections. We are very big, holy, powerful, loving,
very human, and very much like God.

---

*I am as powerful and vast as the sky and as small
and delicate as a little child. I surround and protect the little child in my heart with love so she is
always safe.*

When you listen to yourself and your truths
begin to unfold, do not immediately present
them to the world because discouragement
committees will form to dissuade you.
— Mary Margaret Moore

It takes practice to listen to our intuition and act on it. We have to break our old habit of listening only to what our mind tells us. So it's no wonder we have doubts when we start to listen to our heart.

We often project these doubts onto others. Before we know it, other people are reflecting our doubts and fears back to us, adding their own fears and doubts, and jeopardizing our newfound inspiration. It's a vicious cycle.

We can protect ourselves by imagining that we are surrounded in white light. We can also make it very clear when we want feedback and when we want only support and encouragement for our decisions.

I now listen to my truth. My friends support and encourage me on my spiritual journey. I am safe, secure, and connected.

*There are no more maps, no more creeds,
no more philosophies. From now on in, the
directions come straight from the Divine.*
— Akshara Noor

We live in the Authority Age. In the Authority Age
we often give up all claim to power in exchange for
security. In religion, science, education, government,
or medicine, we're frequently accustomed to some
authority figure knowing all and being in charge.

All of a sudden, along comes AIDS. And years
after those authority figures should have helped to
find a cure, AIDS is still here.

What we have learned is that each of us is on
our own. Although we can support one another and
share love and information, in the end we make
up our own minds. In the end, we decide to be
responsible for ourselves because the authority
figures really don't know what is best for us anyway.

So we turn inward and discover that all real
authority lies there. The source is inside. So is our
connection to all power and security.

*I listen for direction in silence. The voice I hear comes
directly from the Source.*

First of all, a positive attitude is absolutely essential. Be optimistic, hopeful, and cheerful.
— *Tony Petzel, person with AIDS*

We always have control over our attitude. Even when things aren't going the way we want them to and we find ourselves becoming anxious, angry, and afraid, we can change our attitude.

It helps to understand why we're grumpy, afraid, or anxious. Often, it's because we expect our past (especially the unpleasant parts of our past) to relive itself. We feel guilt about what we did, didn't do, thought, didn't think, and we're afraid the past is going to catch up with us.

But the past is over. It has no power over us. The present is here. And we're here in it. In this moment, we can forgive ourselves for all past hurt and harm. We can let go of all guilt and blame. In this moment we can be people who expect only good things to happen. We can be positive.

I am optimistic, hopeful, and cheerful. The past has no power over me. (I forgive the past and let it go.) Wonderful blessings now come my way. Delightful surprises bless me every day.

*A lot of people with AIDS grab the bottle
and head for the grave.*
— *Tom Kaufman, person with AIDS*

One of the hardest situations to deal with is someone else's addiction. It's painful to watch a friend or relative hurt him- or herself day in and day out.

An AIDS diagnosis doesn't make getting clean or sober any easier. For many of us, using alcohol or other drugs was a way to commit slow suicide. Having AIDS just makes it a faster way.

Many of us who are sober now are grateful for the miracle that happened when we turned toward the light and made a decision to live. We're not sure why it happened. It just did.

So we fight against deciding what's best for other people. We try to extend love without judgment. We call in our scattered energies and concentrate on our growth, our sober living, our sanity and health. We trust that our friends are being protected by the same Spirit of the Universe that cares for and watches over us.

Today I pray for all those who still suffer from alcoholism, drug addiction, and all other painful addictions.

The Golden Key: Stop thinking about the difficulty, whatever it is, and think about God instead.

— *Emmet Fox*

Most of us have at least one friend who is always going on about his or her problems. What valuable teachers these friends are. We too have times when we become obsessed with our problems. When they're our problems, they're serious; when our friends are obsessed, we can see it isn't necessary.

How do we stop worrying when we're in the middle of our problems? We move our attention away from them. Some of us use the Serenity Prayer. Others of us meditate or breathe deeply. Or we choose to give our problem to a Higher Power. We use the Golden Key and choose to think only about God and what we imagine God is like: wisdom, truth, beauty, peace, harmony, safety.

The point is, we move our attention away from our difficulties and give them a chance to dissolve.

Peace is my only goal today. When anxious I will turn my attention to the light. I will think only about God as I understand God.

Accept your humanness as well as your
Divinity, totally and without reserve...
And do not shut out the fear, do not deny
anything that seems negative to you.
— *Emmanuel*

Sometimes being human can be depressing. Just when we think we're doing pretty good spiritually speaking, one of our old behaviors resurfaces, or we're filled with feelings we'd rather not have.

But when we deny feelings such as anger, resentment, jealousy, self-pity — part of our humanity — we're being mean to ourselves. Here we are, trying to develop spiritually and live in peace and understanding and we beat ourselves up for being human. But we *are* human.

We are also part of a loving, forgiving, accepting God. As we become more aware of our connection to God, we become more forgiving and accepting of our humanness.

I no longer deny or try to push away any part of myself.
I open my heart and accept my humanness, all of it.
I accept my fear. I accept my anger. It's all part of me.

Sadness is related to the opening of your heart. If you allow yourself to feel sad, especially if you can cry, you will find that your heart opens more and you can feel more love.

— *Shakti Gawain*

Many of us have gone to extremes to prevent ourselves from feeling anything. We've used alcohol and other drugs, sex, other people, food, excitement . . . all to avoid our feelings.

Our logical mind may think sadness is a waste of time. Logical mind can be shaming and criticizing of all our emotions. That's why it's helpful to set logical mind aside and let heart take control. With the guidance of our heart, we can create a safe place for our feelings to surface. We can give ourselves time to feel. We can coax our sadness out and let it rise up for expression.

When we express our sadness, we learn that it isn't the opposite of happiness. Sadness is simply another feeling. And we are most happy when we are able to freely express all our feelings.

I give myself permission to be sad. I allow myself time to cry and express my sadness. I embrace my humanness.

Our fears arise from things we don't confront. Once we are willing to look fully and deeply at the source of a fear, it loses its power.

— *Shakti Gawain*

What am I not willing to look at today? What am I afraid of? When we take time to sit with these questions, we are rewarded with answers.

Maybe we'll learn that we're afraid we won't get our needs met. Maybe we're afraid to look at our addictions. Maybe there are secrets we don't want to think about. Maybe we'll find that we are very sad or tired.

Whatever answer we get, we can either choose to act on it or we can stay in fear. We can face our unfinished business, or we can keep running. The courage we need comes when we ask for help. We don't have to face anything alone.

I am willing to look at all my unfinished business, all my unhealed relationships, all my secrets, all my anxieties. I will start today by asking what needs attention now.

When you ask to be filled with a conscious-
ness that will allow you to love everything
you see and every thought you think, it will
begin to happen.

— *Bartholomew*

I would like to love myself. I want to stop judging myself and other people. I want to stop hating my thoughts and condemning myself. I want to be more loving. What do I do?

Ask. Just ask. This may seem too simple because we're accustomed to creating complicated solutions for living. We're also probably accustomed to doing everything all by ourselves, since many of us aren't used to trusting other people or a Higher Power.

If we really want to change, all we need is a little willingness. We show our willingness when we ask. Once we ask, we can let go of the struggle of trying to control the outcome. The change has already begun; the outcome is assured. As we get in the habit of asking for help, we realize that the world is a friendly, loving place.

Please fill me with the consciousness that allows me
to love everything I see and every thought I think.

What is the family system like where the seed of abuse grows into addiction? It is one where the abuse is denied.
— David Mura

Most of us suffered terribly while growing up. Many of us who have AIDS, or ARC, or are HIV positive, share histories of sexual, physical, or emotional abuse. We often come from alcoholic or other kinds of dysfunctional families. We learned not to talk about how we feel or what's happening to us.

And growing up gay in this society means growing up abused. Like sexually abused children, gay kids are taught to deny the truth about their lives. To avoid the pain of this denial, many of us become addicted to sex, alcohol, or other drugs.

Now, in order to deal with AIDS, we must be free of our addictions and face denial — our own, society's, and our family's. Denial is powerful, but it can't stand up to truth. That's why we create new families where it's safe to express our feelings, safe to talk about abuse, safe to laugh, cry, and be angry, safe to tell the truth.

My feelings set me free. I trust my feelings. I accept and honor the child within me who suffered so much.

When I am able to resist the temptation to judge others, I can see them as teachers of forgiveness in my life, reminding me that I can have peace of mind only when I forgive rather than judge.
— *Gerald Jampolsky*

The more harshly we judge others, the more likely we are to be intolerant of ourselves. It's also likely that behind our judgment is unexpressed anger, hurt, sadness, rage, and fear.

Once we recognize and accept the feelings that cause us to judge, we have a chance to feel them. Once we start feeling, we can confront the truth about what's bothering us. It isn't other people's behavior after all. It's us. Then, forgiveness comes easily and naturally. Then, holding an image of ourselves and the people we judge in the light of our mind's eye, we can imagine our relationships completely healed.

Today I bless all those persons I am tempted to judge. They show me where I am holding anger, and they teach me forgiveness. Today I accept my anger, move with it, and find the forgiveness and peace I need.

Whatever way the game of guilt is played, there must be loss. Someone must lose his innocence that someone else can take it from him, making it his own.
— *A Course in Miracles*

When we feel guilty, we are harmful. We are either self-abusive or we harm others by placing blame on them.

Guilt says we aren't good enough, don't have enough, didn't do enough. Guilt makes us feel as if we've fallen short. To make up for this, we take innocence from another by passing our guilt on to them. But we can choose not to play the game of guilt. We can choose to see the world not as a place of lack but a place of abundance, a place filled with light and love.

Guilt is often subtle, and many of us are so accustomed to living with it that we don't notice it. To become vigilant against guilt we can constantly ask, "Am I being harmless?" When we're being harmless we're living free from guilt and can focus on the world's abundance.

Today I am paying attention. I keep myself harmless because I am innocent and the world is abundant. My gain is my brother's and sister's gain.

I went on a quest to discover what I be-
lieved. If it was life enhancing, I kept it.
If not, I did things to change my belief.
— Will Garcia, person recovering
from AIDS

How do we find out what we believe? Beliefs often hide behind behavior. Patterns in our lives, "the things that always seem to happen to me," can lead us to beliefs or judgments that either set us up as victims of circumstance or empowered actors in life.

We ask ourselves, "What do I believe about myself and the world that leads me to behave this way, and causes these things to happen?" Sometimes the answer comes easily. Sometimes we need help from our friends or professionals. Writing in a journal and meditating help too.

Once we uncover our beliefs, the next step is to replace negative, immune-suppressing beliefs with positive, life-affirming beliefs.

Today I continue my quest to discover what I believe.
I consciously take time to get to know who I am now
and work at letting go of negative ideas about myself.
Today I affirm myself.

I exist as I am, that is enough,
If no other in the world be aware I
*   sit content,*
And if each and all be aware I sit content.
                              — *Walt Whitman*

When we're feeling low and we're afraid we aren't good enough, we can practice self-affirmation — active, positive self-acceptance. We affirm, "I am what I am."

Daily doses of "I am what I am" therapy is an antidote to the poison of perfectionism. We grew up believing that approval depended on what we did. And we could never do enough, good enough. So today, we still worry that we aren't acceptable, that we are never finished, presentable, good enough.

As we practice self-acceptance, we let go of that old anxiety. The more we tell ourselves we are fine just the way we are, the less we worry we have about what others think. We become less self-conscious, more relaxed. We discover that people like us just the way we are.

All day long, whether I am conscious of it or not, I will receive positive messages that say, "I am perfect today in every way."

It is a common experience that a problem difficult at night is resolved in the morning after the committee of sleep has worked on it.

— *John Steinbeck*

Each of us has a great problem solving resource: our internal guide, our inner committee. One way to use our guides is to directly and specifically discuss our situation, problem, or dilemma with them before we fall asleep. We can ask that, through our dreams, they help us resolve our problems.

It's a little like using the worry dolls Guatemalan children use. They keep tiny dolls in a box by their bed. At night they give each of their problems to a doll and ask that doll to worry about it for them, so they can get a good night's sleep.

Anyway, in the morning, before we get out of bed, we try to recall our dreams, and listen to our feelings; we get a committee report. Then, throughout the day, we'll be amazed at our understanding, clarity, and peace.

I turn all my problems over to my inner committee, and I go free.

If the total integrated system of mind, body and emotions, which constitutes the whole person, is not working in the direction of health, then purely physical interventions may not succeed.
— Carl and Stephanie Simonton

Many of us have been out of balance. We've ignored our emotions and neglected our bodies. Healing for us means attending to all our needs — emotional, intellectual, spiritual, physical. If we ignore any one part of ourselves for too long, all parts suffer.

We need to make sure our whole self is working together as a team. If emotionally we want to stay sick in order to get attention, then, the attention we give our emotional self may be the most important thing we can do to heal physically.

The point is to make sure that all parts of us are pulling for the same thing, that all our needs are being met. Hugs are just as important as vitamins.

I expand my consciousness to surround and include my whole self. I attend to all my needs — emotional, mental, spiritual, and physical. I stand united, facing the light.

The map is not the territory.
— *Alfred Korzybski*

Talking about God is not the same as experiencing God. Professing belief in some kind of Higher Power and actually experiencing the presence of that holy spirit are two different matters.

Many of us turned away from organized religion because we thought religion confused the map (dogma and theory) with the territory (serenity, peace, wholeness).

Reading and talking about spirituality are important, but at a certain point we have to be quiet and listen. We have to allow the experience to happen. Silent prayer and meditation open us to experience. So can walking alone outside, listening to music, running, yoga.

Whatever we do, the point is that we not take our spiritual practice, our dogma, too seriously. Our beliefs, our creeds, our activities are only tools, maps that point us toward the real thing.

Today I will sit in silent prayer and meditation. I will lightly hold my maps, my creeds, my thinking, and my spirituality. I know a holy spirit is present in my heart without them.

We want to create hope for the person and acceptance in the hearts of the people. We must give hope, always hope and remove the bitterness that is harming them when they are being avoided by everyone.
— *Mother Teresa on AIDS*

No drug is as powerful as hope. It has no toxic side effects and you can't overdose on it. Hope is available to all of us right now without Food and Drug Administration approval, and it's free.

Hope opens a space for miracles to happen. Miracles are the natural result of hope. Supporting hope are trust and faith. If our hope is fading, maybe we are relying on ourselves too much and need to place our trust in a Higher Power, maybe we need to have faith that we're always protected and loved.

And though we can't make other people accept us and we can't control how others deal with AIDS, we can be forgiving and hope that they find loving acceptance for themselves.

As we concentrate on accepting ourselves, we will find that acceptance reflected back to us in everyone we meet.

My hope is contagious; I spread it wherever I go. I forgive and let go of all bitterness and regret. I trust that I am always cared for and loved.

i thank You God for this most amazing
day; for the leaping greenly spirits of trees
and a blue true dream of sky; and
   for everything
which is natural which is infinite which
   is yes.

— e. e. cummings

Today I will notice. If possible, I will walk outside and look for dandelions and new green buds on bushes and trees. I will look for blackbirds building nests and robins digging worms. I will look at the clouds and try to name the color of the sky. I will notice the color of light and the shadows made by buildings, clotheslines, and fences.

Today I will listen, really listen to the sounds made by birds, traffic, church bells, and construction workers. I will try to hear children laughing, dogs barking, cars honking, and the wind.

Today I will hug a tree and hold my hand against the ground. I will notice how my skin feels when the cool breeze blows against the back of my neck. I will caress my naked body, walk barefoot in the grass, and enjoy the warm sun on my face. Today is my day to pay attention and give thanks.

I give thanks for all my senses. They are all I need to know God.

Be willing to accept the shadows that walk across the sun.

— *Emmanuel*

Our difficulties have been our teachers. We know that. Yet we often have a hard time accepting that this is true for other people. We forget that everyone is on a path — not just us.

When we see other people suffering, it's hard to accept it, just as it's difficult to view AIDS as anything but a tragedy. But AIDS is a teacher for all of us. We're learning things such as how to accept love, how to give unconditional love, how to trust, how to die, how to live, how to stand up and be empowered, how to let go, how to surrender, how to ask for help.

AIDS also teaches us about our spiritual essence, that we are connected to, united with, all living things. And so, we walk in the light, unafraid of the shadows. We know that without our shadows none of us would be aware of the light.

Even when I don't understand and my belief is small, I am open to the idea that all is right in the world.

I've discovered I'm a strong and capable person. I can handle almost anything except being alone with this.
— *Keith Gann, person with AIDS*

In the midst of activity, even in the middle of support groups and meetings, we can be alone. We can go through the motions but not reach out.

This is why we need to find time to talk to at least one person about our feelings, fears, and hopes. If we don't, we're probably not getting enough support. At the same time, if we don't take time to be with ourselves, we're also denying ourselves powerful support.

To be intimate with another person and with our self, we have to be honest. We must be willing to trust, to risk, and be vulnerable. Many of us are so afraid of being discounted, criticized, or not listened to, that we don't trust or take the risk.

The worst that can happen is that we'll be hurt or disappointed. We have all survived hurt and disappointment. But we may not survive being isolated with AIDS. Reaching out to others is worth the risk.

Today I pray for the willingness to open up and be honest with myself and at least one other person. I will take a risk. I will do whatever I need to do today to be supported.

You are swimming in deep water without allowing fear and panic to cause you to drown.

— *David Bennett*

Those of us affected by AIDS have become good at keeping our heads when people around us are losing theirs. We don't give ourselves enough credit for it either. We're doing more than surviving crazy times; we're growing stronger, wiser, warmer, and more loving every day.

We're beginning to see that our real struggle is with fear. So we try to stay away from people who spread fear, stay out of rooms that are filled with fear, and avoid the media that promotes fear.

We can also make a friend of fear. When we feel fear is present, we can simply sit still and find the place in our body where it is most acute. Then we can surround this place with loving energy summoned from the rest of our body, energy that we have in abundance.

Today I pray for the courage to turn around and calmly face my fears. Even when fear is present, I know that I am not fear, I am love.

People have been curing themselves of incurable diseases for centuries. Now we're doing it with AIDS.
— *Tony Petzel, person with AIDS*

As Louise Hay, the author of *You Can Heal Your Life,* says, incurable simply means you have to go inside to find the cure. And it is happening. It's happening all across the country. Regularly now, many people with AIDS are rejecting the statistics, ignoring the doomsayers, and recovering.

After all, if our bodies can perform miracles like heal a broken bone, or make new skin, or repair muscles and tissue, they can also perform the miracle of repairing a broken immune system.

Of course, healing the body may not be the most important activity for some of us; healing our body may not be where we will learn the most. If our body doesn't respond the way we think it should, it doesn't mean we are failing. It may mean our growth, our healing, is happening on another level.

We receive our lessons individually packaged, custom made, slightly different from the next person's. We can't compare how we're doing with another person. Life is not a competition.

I gratefully accept all my lessons, however they come packaged.

July

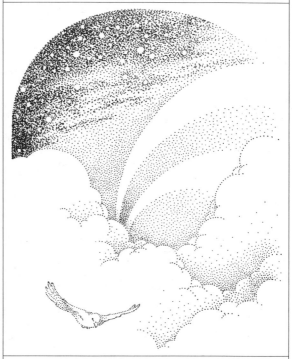

I love moving from one emotion to another. I love and appreciate the full rainbow of my emotions.

*You know what makes you sing, what
makes you dance and laugh and love. But
if you do not ask yourself what it is you
know, you will go on listening to others and
change will not come because you will not
hear your own truth.*

— *Bartholomew*

If we were suddenly given a test about current
events, many of us would know the answers. If we
were given a pop quiz on AIDS, we'd probably do
even better. But we probably wouldn't do well if
we were given a test about ourselves: What do you
most like to do? What makes you happy?

Many of us have buried answers to these questions deep in our minds. It's time to uncover them
and get to know who we are. If we're not acting
on what makes us sing, dance, and love, we're
probably acting out someone else's reality. Getting
to know ourselves is new territory, and it can be
confusing and frustrating. Panic may set in.

That's when a simple prayer such as "Please help
me sit still and listen" helps a lot.

*Today I will start a written list of the things that make
me happy. I will begin introducing myself to myself.
If I become afraid, I will pray for help and remember
to breathe.*

Guilt is the little engine that drives compulsive behavior.

— *George Marcelle*

We all know the feeling. When we were little and did something really wrong we got a big sinking feeling in our stomach. Later, we felt guilty just for being who we were. For many of us, guilt has been our constant companion.

There's a lot of guilt surrounding AIDS, guilt we need to face and get rid of it as soon as possible. First we need to stop running and admit to ourselves all those things that we've been denying. We need to finally call everything by its right name and bring into the open everything we feel guilty about. Everything.

Then, it helps to tell our story to someone we trust. Once we have admitted it all, we can let go of it. We can forgive ourselves and know that we have been forgiven for all we think we have done.

In the process we learn that we are and have always been innocent in God's eyes.

I forgive myself totally. I am an innocent child of God.

And acceptance is the answer to all my problems today. . . I can find no serenity until I accept that person, place, thing, or situation as being exactly the way it is supposed to be at this moment.
— *Alcoholics Anonymous*

Acceptance does not mean suffering. Suffering puts walls around pain, closes in on it, and tries to change it. Acceptance allows pain to move. Suffering, like self-pity, holds on to disturbing thoughts and keeps them hostage. Acceptance lets them pass.

Suffering despairs and curses fate behind God's back. Acceptance stands at the top of the hill, faces the wind, throws back his shoulders and screams. Acceptance allows energy to move.

Accepting "that person, place, or thing" doesn't mean we have to like it. We don't have to like our illnesses or situations. We don't have to be quiet about them either. It's okay to make a fuss, even a big fuss. Acceptance means letting energy move. It means we're alive.

Acceptance is the answer to all my problems today. Energy moves around me, past me, through me. I am changing.

If you have never loved yourself, never really loved yourself, gently and unconditionally, now is the time to do that.
— Max Navarre, person with AIDS

AIDS puts things in perspective. It asks us to slow down and do all the self-loving, healing things we've been putting off. One thing we can do is forgive ourselves for any pain we've caused to others, to the earth, to God, and to ourselves. If we could have done anything differently, we would have.

The next thing we can do is tell ourselves about our love. Out loud. We can talk to ourselves and say, "I love you. I really love you." (It sounds corny, but these are words we've needed to hear for a long time, words we can never hear enough.)

Words start us in the right direction. Action carries us forward. We need to do the things that give us joy. Whatever they are, from walking in the woods, to playing the piano, to calling up a friend, to going to a ball game, or watching movies and eating popcorn.

Today, I commit to being kind to my mind, my body, and my emotions. I commit to treating myself tenderly and with loving devotion.

*You are here to see where you are in Light
and also to find the residual areas of
    darkness
that are determined to sabotage the Light.*
                                — *Emmanuel*

When an area of our lives give us pain —
relationships, health, money, sex, alcohol or other
drugs — there is a part of us blocking the light: an
attitude, a belief, judgment, some form of fear.

When we acknowledge this and become willing
to honestly look at ourselves, we begin a motion
toward positive change. We needn't wait until the
pain caused by our old behavior is unbearable. With
a little bit of willingness, we can marshal the courage
we need to honestly look at our lives right now.
If we are willing, we will be able to see that we make
our own shadows.

Once we are aware of the fears that cause our
pain, we can change. We can take responsibility for
our lives without blame, guilt, or shame.

---

*Grant me the courage to look at my life honestly and
with compassion.*

Only accumulated emotional pain and misinformation stand in the way of our loving ourselves and each other fully and without shame, pretense or reluctance. We must therefore encourage each other in the natural process of crying, raging, trembling, laughing, yawning and talking, through which our hurts are healed.
— *Christopher Spence*

Encouragement begins at home. The more we encourage ourselves to express our feelings, the more genuine will be the encouragement we give our friends. When we give ourselves permission to cry, rage, laugh, and talk, we become encouragers of emotion. Unafraid of our own emotions, we aren't afraid of our friends' emotions either. Patient with ourselves, we are patient with others.

One to one, in groups, big and small, we encourage healing. We do our part to create an atmosphere in which we and our friends are allowed to go through changes.

I consciously move toward loving myself and my friends, "fully and without shame, pretense or reluctance." I support myself and others in laughing, crying, raging, trembling, yawning, talking. We dance together in the sunlight.

Children have a magical ability not to place limits on their thinking and dreaming. Anything and everything is possible for those who believe, and children understand this better than anyone.
— *Susan Smith Jones, Ph.D.*

What are the limits we place on our thinking and dreaming? What boundaries do we place on what we can believe, have, do, be, want, become?

Hard questions. It may help to try and remember when we stopped dreaming big. When did our imagination begin to fade and our childhood end? When did words like "should," "can't," and "but" enter our lives?

If we sit with these questions for a while and don't get clear answers, that's all right. We don't need the specifics right now; we need the feelings. We need to recover the feelings that surround our lost dreams. They are part of us. Reclaimed, they make us whole.

As we recover the lost parts of ourselves we can make a decision to become believers again. We can gently decide that we were wrong to limit our dreams. Now it's time to recover our lost dreams and create new dreams.

Today I reclaim the dreaming and believing wisdom that was mine long ago.

*Both the Stone of Harmony and the Stone
of Uncaring can be the Drums that Set
the Rings of Water Into Motion Within the
Dance of the Medicine Lake.... If
the People Care for One Another, then the
Rings of this Dance are Harmonious.*
— *Hyemeyohosts Storm*

Every day, what we do ripples throughout our
world — our Medicine Lake. Every day, we have a
choice. We can choose to carry the Stone of
Uncaring or the Stone of Harmony.

Before AIDS, many of us didn't think we had a
choice and didn't think it mattered much anyway.
We thought what we did and who we were didn't
affect anyone else. We were wrong. When we oper-
ated out of fear, loneliness, isolation, and low
self-esteem, we dropped a Stone of Uncaring that
touched everyone. AIDS is teaching us that we make
a difference.

Each time we reach out to help or allow someone to help us, we add to the reservoir of hope,
we make a difference. We say, I am one of the people who care.

*Today I choose the stone of harmony. I care for myself
and I care for other people. Today I dance with the
people who care.*

Thus, with a child or the child grown into an adult, a therapist listens to the pain behind the words, behind the official or accepted version of the past, the white-wash of a happy or "normal" childhood.
— David Mura

Each of us can listen carefully to the pain behind the words of others, whether we're hearing about someone's childhood or about how things are now. If we're willing to listen, people will talk. It takes being quiet longer than normal, and giving our full attention to the other person for ten minutes, thirty minutes, an hour.

In that time, we don't talk about ourselves or worry what we're going to say next. We only ask questions and encourage our friend to talk. And we try to really hear what our friend is saying and feeling. When we do, we will begin to understand how it is for someone else. We will be compassionate.

If we're willing to listen to others, we'll be more willing to let others listen to us. We all need to be heard beyond, "How are you?" "I am fine."

I listen to the feeling behind the words. And I let others in on what I'm feeling too. One by one we share our truths.

Spiritual growth is more of the nature of proceeding from hunch to hunch than from conclusion to conclusion.

— *John Fortunato*

Faith and trust in some kind of Higher Power can grow like a tree from a seed. It doesn't have to leap into our lives full grown.

All that faith needs is a small opening, a crack to slip through. We don't have to be sure; we don't have to believe with all our mind and heart. A hunch will do, a simple hunch that there is more to this world than what we might think.

When we allow for the possibility that there is some force beyond our ego and we whisper, "I can't do this alone, please help me," change begins. The seed takes root in our heart. That's all we need for a miracle.

Each time we follow our hunches or listen to our intuition, we water and fertilize our faith. Our trust grows stronger and the world seems safer. And even if we don't have clear, logical explanations for everything, it doesn't matter. We're living from our heart and that feels right.

I cultivate my intuition and watch my faith grow. I shine my attention on my hunches, like the sun shines on newly sprouted plants.

You cannot read the future from a path-
ology report or a blood test. Individuals are
not statistics.

— *Bernie Siegel*

Because we know so little about AIDS, we reach for information, any information. We sometimes rely too heavily on test results or statistics to give us a measure of certainty in an uncertain world. These numbers make us feel like we have some control.

Yet, an overemphasis on statistics and test results can make us feel hopeless. Many of us have decided our lives are over because of a positive HIV anti-body test or a low T-cell count.

We've been terrorized by dubious tests and statistics for long enough. It's time to stop letting numbers and lab reports limit our options.

The universe is abundant, and its blessings are available to us all. The future is made today. The universe is not predictable. It is lively, raucous, wild, and open. It cannot be contained within the neat parameters of statistics or test results. And neither can we.

I turn away from constricting statistics that try to explain away my life. I open to the limitless abundance of a universe that is unfolding at my feet.

*Although my spiritual practice is far from
consistent, I know that God is directing my
life, and that peace of God is my goal.*
— *Gerald Jampolsky*

God is directing my life. Peace of God is my goal.
What a powerful affirmation. When we affirm that
God is directing our life, we decide to let go of our
will and accept God's will. We decide that we don't
have to control everything and everyone. As we let
go, we begin to trust other people, events, ourselves,
the world.

Even if our belief in God is thin or nonexistent,
we can all feel an increasing sense of adventure as
we begin to work out our understanding of what
spirituality means. Our prejudices against "religious
people" slip away and we begin to explore the
exciting world of the spirit.

However unlikely or unpromising our beginning
is, we can all nurture and build a faith in a Power
greater than ourselves. As we do, we learn to surrender control of our lives to that force, however
we understand it, by whatever name we call it.

*I accept my deep, personal spirituality. I nurture and
support my spirit nature. I trust the creative spirit of
the universe. Peace of God is my only goal today.*

Take heed, be quiet, do not fear.
                    — Isaiah 7:4

Even when we know how important and satisfying prayer and meditation are, we often don't take time to pray and meditate, which can be the perfect set-up for a personal scolding and shaming. So we need to be careful. Punishing ourselves for not being good to ourselves is pretty silly.

Our ego plays it both ways. It tells us how important it is to be quiet and meditate. Then it raises fears such as: I can't do this; I'll fail. There's nothing out there anyway; I'm not a true spiritual person after all.

We do have a choice though; we can avoid the traps our ego sets for us. We can simply sit still, breathe deep, exhale, pause. Breathe again, exhale, pause. Breathe, exhale, pause. . . . When thoughts arise, we bless them and let them pass.

The more we sit quietly, the more receptive we become. When we aren't busy worrying, our fears disappear.

I am quiet. My heart is strong. My fears are gone. I am listening.

*My disease has been a demanding teacher
that has guided me — sometimes with a
heavy hand — toward what I need to do.*
— *Tom O'Connor, person with ARC*

There's an adage that goes, "When the student
is ready, the teacher appears." (For many of us, AIDS
is our teacher.) Good teachers not only help us learn
new things, they also help us let go of old ideas
and old behaviors.

Maybe we need to let go of dependence on
alcohol, other drugs, or cigarettes. Maybe letting go
of negative ideas of how we think of ourselves is
what we need. Maybe it's time to deal with family
issues and let go of resentment and rage.

Maybe it's time to let go of some deep sadness
and grief, to sit still for a long time and cry or scream
as loudly as we can.

If we are open to listening and learning from our
teachers, we will know what our next healing step
needs to be. We will lighten our load because we
will know what to set free.

*Divine Spirit, take away all those things that stand
in the way of my usefulness to you and others.*

I worked with the idea of safety, that I was constantly safe. I began to use fear rather than let fear use me. And as I began to live my life, my body began to come alive.
— *George Melton, person recovering from AIDS*

The belief that we aren't safe is the basis for most of our anxiety, tension, stress, and disease. When we identify only with our bodies, we become afraid. AIDS is good at bringing out this fear.

But there is another way of looking at the world. It starts with believing that we are more than our bodies. We are also spirit; we are connected to and part of the source of all life. The Spirit of the Universe is our protector and friend. We need never be afraid.

Yet, until we learn to live without fear, we can use our fears. They teach us where we need to heal. We can follow fear to its source and listen to its message, discovering old hurts that need to be cared for, old emotions that need permission to be expressed. Then, all the places where fear lives we can touch with love.

I am more than my body. I bless my fears; they teach me how to heal.

*. . . the need is to recognize that the patient
is the healer — not the doctor.*
— *Norman Cousins*

Many of us are well-trained for the role of sub-servient patient. We were trained to believe that other people and outside circumstances can deter-mine our health and happiness, and that doctors make us well.

But that attitude doesn't work with AIDS. And so many of us have started taking responsibility for our healing. We have recognized that choices exist and that we make them happen.

We're understanding that all healing happens in-side our bodies and that we can communicate with our bodies to help our healing. So we call back any energy and power that we may have left in our doctor's office and we begin to attend to ourselves. We make choices based on what feels right, based on our own truth.

And we thank our doctors and other healers for their help; they are our peers and friends. And we know that each of us is a doctor of divine healing.

I am a powerful healer because I am connected to the one source of all healing and love.

Those of us who are not sick and are watching people who are sick, feel tremendously helpless.

— Mark Jacobs

Many of us think we should be doing more and doing it better. We feel guilty. We're afraid people are judging us and we don't measure up. Some of us feel guilty because we're healthy while our friends are sick.

We need to throw all that guilt out the window. While we're at it, let's dump as much blame, fear of punishment, and shame as we can. None of these negative emotions help us.

In place of guilt, we substitute unconditional love and 100 percent acceptance for the way we are, healthy or ill, AIDS diagnosed or not.

In place of helplessness, we can substitute helpfulness. All of us can do something — from giving care, to stuffing envelopes, to praying, to loving ourselves and our friends. All of us can carry a message of hope and unconditional love.

I trust that just as I am always at the right place at the right time, so are my friends. Just as I have a Higher Power watching over me, so do they.

Namaste. I salute the Divinity in you which salutes the divinity in me.

— *Yoga greeting*

Many of us grew up believing we are each separate, isolated, and alone. We learned to live in fear, afraid other people were going to hurt us, afraid there wasn't enough love to go around.

There is another way to view the world. It says we all are one. No one is separate. We're all made up of the same stuff, all part of God. When I look at you I can choose to be afraid or I can choose to see myself reflected in you. Then, giving and receiving are the same, there is no lack, and I need not be afraid.

When we feel alone and small, we have chosen to believe in a world of separation and fear. We can change our minds and choose a world of unity and love. Every person we meet today we can silently salute with the greeting: *Namaste.* We can also place the palms of our hands together, hold them over our heart, and bow slightly to ourselves in the mirror. Namaste.

You are part of God and so am I. Namaste.

*You are so much more than you believe
you are.*

— Bartholomew

We tend to identify with our body. I am this person who weighs 150 pounds, stands 5 feet 8 inches
tall, is 39 years old. . . . I am this person who has
AIDS. . . . I have an AIDS-related condition. . . .
I test positive to the HIV virus.

When we identify only with our body, the condition of our body determines our feelings and
attitudes — whether we are happy, peaceful, anxious,
fearful, angry, or depressed. When we identify only
with our body, we walk in a small, narrow world.

Is it possible that we have made a mistake in our
identity? Perhaps, in addition to our body, we are
also a powerful field of energy connected to other
powerful fields of energy, connected to the source
of all energy.

Perhaps, inside each of us is a vast pool of love,
an ocean of memory, and a space big enough to
include the world. If this is true, we no longer need
to feel lonely, shameful, or afraid. We are much
more than our bodies.

*Today I will imagine what I am beyond the bound-
aries of my body. I will let myself imagine without
having to believe.*

Do not inflict your will.
Just give love.
The soul will take that love
and put it where it can best be used.
— *Emmanuel*

Sometimes the hardest thing about loving people with AIDS is letting go, especially if we tend to be caretakers. We want others to do their healing our way.

Wanting someone to do it our way presumes that we know what's best for that person. It also presumes that what's happening in that person's life isn't for the best. How do we know?

Our anxiety about another's behavior is often a projection of our own fear. We don't trust. We fear that unless we have tight control of the world around us, the sky will fall.

So if we are anxious about how another person is living his or her life, it may be a sign that we need to turn our attention to ourselves. We need to trust that the powers at work in our lives are also at work in theirs. We are most helpful to others when we trust, relax, and know that our lives and their lives are unfolding according to plan.

Help me let go of my need to control. Teach me to trust.

Funding a will through action, yet un-attached to outcomes, remaining mindful that all you can really do is stay out of your own way and let the Will of Heaven flow through you — these are among the hallmarks of the Spiritual Warrior.

— *Ralph Blum*

When we are attached to results, when we want everything to go "our way," we manipulate people. People don't like to be manipulated, so they rebel. Then we try harder. Our anxiety builds. We're afraid that if the outcome isn't the one we want, it will be bad for us. Because, of course, we believe we live in a hostile world.

We need to start believing that the world is safe, and that the outcomes the universe thinks up will be better than what we wanted.

Then we go about our business. We take action. We visualize outcomes. But this time, we hold on to our images loosely. We keep our minds open to new possibilities, trusting the universe to provide us with just the right experiences.

I am a Spiritual Warrior. I take positive action yet I stay flexible, open to new possibilities. I trust the universe and surrender to its will.

. . .one of the benefits of their illness was that they could no longer ignore their true needs. The illness permitted them to. . . express their feelings and go about meeting their needs openly and directly.
— *Carl and Stephanie Simonton*

In the past, many of us acted as though we didn't need anything from anyone. Of course, that wasn't true. We needed to be touched, held, loved, appreciated, listened to, cared for. But we didn't know how to ask for it, so we acted out inappropriately, tried to get our needs met indirectly, became caretakers of other people or abused alcohol, other drugs, sex, or food.

Now, as individuals and as a community, we're learning how to touch and be touched, how to listen, how to talk, how to be emotionally honest. AIDS is teaching us how to accept our humanity.

And we are teaching each other that we don't have to get sick to get our emotional needs met. When we ask others for what we need clearly and directly, it's easier for them to respond.

Today I will make a list of my true needs — emotional, intellectual, spiritual, physical. I will make another list of ways to get those needs met.

(i who have died am alive again today,
and this is the sun's birthday; this is
*   the birth*
day of life and of love and wings; and of
*   the gay*
great happening illimitably earth)
                              — e. e. cummings

Every day, when we wake up, we are reborn.
Everything is new, not an unbroken chain of yesterday and tomorrow. We wake up, step out of our
dream world, and are given today. Not this week,
this month, this year, or "the rest of my life." Just
today. A nice, manageable chunk of time.

We can do all sorts of things "just today." We can
be clean and sober, just today. We can have a positive attitude, today. We can believe in ourselves,
today. Today we can be forgiving. Today we can
choose peace instead of conflict. Today we can
imagine that everything we eat makes our cells jump
with energy; every breath we take charges our blood.

We can decide that just for today we will smile
at people. Today love will ripple out from us in
all directions. Just for today, we will walk the earth
in peace.

Today I celebrate the sun's birthday. I celebrate my
rebirth. Break out the balloons.

We shall need to raise our eyes toward perfection, and be ready to walk in that direction. It will seldom matter how haltingly we walk. The only question will be, "Are we ready?"

— *Bill Wilson*

AIDS is telling us to make our lives everything we want them to be. Now. So, what do I want my life to be? What kind of person am I at my core? And what's the difference between how I'm living my life now and that ideal? What parts of my character, what habits stand in the way of me expressing my true, creative self?

When we start to answer questions like these, it's easy to fall into the "oh what's the use" trap. There seems to be too much to do.

Gratefully, we don't have to "do" it. We only need to be willing to have our problems, obstacles, habits, character defects removed. We only need to be ready to let go of all those things that aren't us. Becoming a perfect "me" is a worthy goal. When we reach it isn't as important as the fact that we're walking in that direction.

I am ready to let go of all those things that keep me from becoming my true, creative, perfect self. Please take them from me.

*And then he gave a very long sigh and said,
"I wish Pooh were here. It's so much more
friendly with two."*
— *Piglet, from* Winnie the Pooh
by A.A. Milne

Many of us know that our recovery from alcoholism or other addictions began when we made contact with other recovering people. We weren't alone anymore. Others understood what we were going through and that made it bearable. Life became more friendly.

AIDS works the same way. It's just too lonesome to deal with AIDS alone. Whether we're a person who has AIDS, the mother or father of a person with AIDS, the lover of a person with AIDS, or at high risk, we all need support.

AIDS is fightable if we do it together, which means reaching out and picking up the phone and talking. It means asking for help. It means going to group support meetings, and staying in touch with friends and new people we meet. It means taking steps out of isolation into community. Until, sooner or later, connecting with other people becomes natural again.

My life is more friendly now that I am taking more risks and reaching out to others.

All goes onward and outward...and
  nothing collapses.
And to die is different from what anyone
  supposed, and luckier.
— *Walt Whitman*

We have their word on it. Poets, people who
return from near death experiences, and great
spiritual teachers all agree: death is not such
a bad deal.

Facing the possibility of exploding out into the
next life can make this life more interesting. Facing
death makes living more immediate, current, and
important. It brings us into the present.

The point is, if we aren't afraid to die, why be
afraid to live? Yet, sometimes we are. We're afraid
to take risks in relationships, in career, in our treatments. We're afraid of our spirituality and creativity.

We need to find where we're acting out of fear,
where we are holding back from living fully. Then,
without denying our fear, or being ashamed of it,
we need to ask ourselves if it's valid, if it makes
sense. After all, if we're no longer afraid to die, we
don't need to be afraid to live.

*Today I will imagine that, when I die, I will explode
into new life. I will also imagine exploding into new
life right now, without dying.*

In abused children, one often finds a troubling self-assurance, an adult like manner that seems to deny any suffering or turmoil. This act of self-assurance protects the child from what would happen if the child were to feel the terror, rage, sadness and shame of abuse. It is a tool of survival.
— David Mura

As children, many of us learned how to hide our feelings and shut down emotionally. Later, we may have used alcohol or other drugs to keep from feeling. Now, as we begin to unravel our past, as we step out of the fog, we run the risk of going back to the bottle, the needle, or whatever we were using to numb ourselves.

We don't have to flee into oblivion. We aren't children anymore. We aren't alone either. With help from our friends, from our Higher Power, from therapy, we can finally experience some of the feelings we've been avoiding for so long.

When we were children, we had no choice. Now we do. We can choose to experience our feelings. We can step out of emotional numbness.

God help me let go of survival tools that no longer serve me. Restore me to intimate contact with myself and all my emotions.

As a tree grows tall, the roots grow deep
and strong and wide. Let your humanness
become part of your strength.
                              — Emmanuel

We all need affection, support, encouragement,
food, clothing, shelter. When our needs are being
met, we feel safe enough to express our feelings.
But when our needs aren't met, or we deny our
needs, we don't feel safe enough to express our feelings. We shut down.

To grow, we must begin to accept our humanness. The more we own up to who we are — with
humility and acceptance — the stronger we become.
Each time we ask for what we need, we sink our
roots deeper and wider. Every time we express our
feelings, honestly and directly, we grow in love.

To grow spiritually, we need to be rooted in our
humanness. Like the branches of a tree, our spirit
seeks the light and feeds our roots, our humanness.
Our roots send up nourishment and strength and
feed our spirit.

I imagine that I am a tree. Down through the base
of my spine I send my roots deep and wide into the
earth. I send my branches to the sky. I am a growing,
breathing, vital, spiritual human being.

Who sees his Lord
Within every creature,
Deathlessly dwelling
Amidst the mortal:
That man sees truly.

— *Bhagavad-Gita*

Sometimes, seeing clearly is only a matter of slowing down to look more closely. While going about our business it's easy to miss the essence of other people and things. We miss that which is larger, beyond appearance. We miss God (or whatever words we use to name the unnameable) in other people.

But if we do look closely, with all our senses, we will feel a connection, a thread running between us and others, a wave of energy moving back and forth. If we do look closely, we will recognize a relative, a kin. More closely still, and we see ourselves.

That's why feeling hopeless and lonely come from believing in the illusion of separateness. We can learn to see through the illusion by slowing down long enough to look more closely at the people, animals, plants all around us.

Help me look carefully and see the truth. Help me recognize You in all Your earthly disguises. Help me acknowledge You in me.

When aids is over we're going to look back and say that, because of aids, we learned how to love ourselves and each other.
— Louie Nassaney, person with AIDS

When AIDS is over. What a powerful notion. For many of us, the idea that AIDS will end is hard to imagine. But the end of AIDS is worth thinking about. It's important to see ourselves as happy, healthy, productive, and free from the constant concern about AIDS.

Our lives will never be restored to how they were before AIDS. We are all changed. Society is changed. Medicine and healing are changed. We have become a more empowered, loving, united community — not just those of us who are gay, but all of us who have been touched by AIDS.

We don't have to wait until the end of AIDS though. Right now we can visualize our lives, happy, healthy, productive, and free from the constant concern about AIDS. Healed and well.

Because of AIDS, I am more loving, accepting, sincere, and hopeful than I was before. I am intimate with people in a way I didn't know was possible before. I have learned to love and accept myself totally.

The teacher is within, so you have to learn to be still . . . you have to learn to live your life so that you are listening within, no matter what you are doing.

— *Bartholomew*

To become acquainted with the teacher within, we need to spend time alone. We need to give our inner teacher the time and space to make his or her presence known to us.

We may also need help from other people. They can help us learn how to meditate, how to listen and we can join with other people and our mutual seeking can help us find what we're looking for.

Each of us can find the outside support we need, even if we have to get it over the telephone or through the mail.

Making the change from running through life with our spiritual ears plugged to listening requires only a little willingness and a little practice. Our teachers are waiting to help us.

My teacher has always been here with me. I knew it all along. I love my teacher.

August

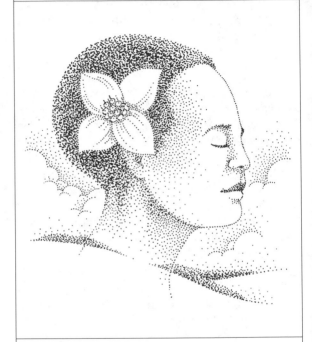

In quiet meditation, like a flower in a field, I turn toward the light. The light is sweet and I am safe and warm.

*Settle for nothing less than what you truly
desire, and do not be afraid to ask for what
you feel will bring you joy and fulfillment.*
— Emmanuel

Many of us are afraid to ask for what we truly
want. Most of the time we don't even know what
we want. We're afraid of the question.

Today is the day to ask, "What do I really want?
What will make me most happy?" Today is the day
to sit down and make a list of what we want.
Anything goes as long as we are as honest and
thoughtful as possible. No one else needs to see
what we write.

The point is to push at the walls of our imagination and to be as open, generous, and creative as
we can. The point is to stretch.

Once we've made our list and are comfortable
with it, we come to the next step. We ask out loud
for what we want. As we ask, we add, "This or
something better now manifests for me, for my
good, and for the good of all concerned."

---

*I am expanding the boundaries of my dreams. I want
to go as far as I can in this lifetime. I want to be happy,
joyous, and free.*

The human and the divine, the solar and the lunar, day and night, conscious and unconscious, female and male, adult and child, all worlds are actually one, dimensions of one another. . . . The knowledge of this. . . is the fruit of wholeness.
— *Rachel V.*

Like King Arthur's knight, Percivale, each of us is on a journey, a quest. Like him, we too sometimes need a crisis to push us out into the world, to start us moving down the path of self-discovery.

AIDS can be the push we need, the crisis that forces us to discover our spirituality, to recognize our divinity, and to accept our humanness. In our search for our Holy Grail, we learn that darkness and light are part of the same world, and fear is the flip side of faith. We learn that the body and soul are not divided, and death does not end life.

I now know that what I seek I already have. I already have love in my heart, and I already am one with all things.

Eventually I lost interest in trying to control my life, to make things happen in a way that I thought I wanted them to be. I began to practice surrendering to the universe and finding out what "it" wanted me to do.

— *Shakti Gawain*

Thinking back on our lives to those experiences that have been life-changing and to those opportunities that were most wonderful, we probably will discover that they all just sort of happened to us. They weren't part of our plan.

Knowing this, why is it so hard to let go and trust the universe? Maybe it's because of how we were raised. We were encouraged to be rational. Intuition and daydreaming were discouraged. We learned fear from people who were afraid.

That was then and this is now. Now we can support our daydreaming and listen to our intuition. Now we know that what the "universe wants me to do" is always the highest expression of my own true self. Now we know that God's idea of a good time is pretty wonderful indeed.

The universe communicates to me through my intuition. I trust its guidance and act on its direction.

It is a stupefying thing, grief. It comes over me sharply, at unexpected moments, in the middle of me cooking something he would have liked, or hearing music he enjoyed. . . . I stop, I cry; I let the feeling feel me. And then I do the hardest thing: I put aside the guilt I feel about surviving and being well, and continue with my life.
— *Doug Federhart*

Grief is a feeling with a life of its own. It surfaces according to its own schedule. If we are too busy for grief, if we deny it, we cut ourselves off from our emotions and we become smaller. Our grief gets smaller too — tighter, more compact, more intense, explosive.

It's best not to get too busy for grief. It's best to be open and expansive and available for all our feelings, including our grief. They won't take up our whole lives or all our time, and there won't be more pain than we can bear.

If we give our feelings time and space to express themselves, there will also be time and space enough for us to go on with the rest of our lives.

Today I let my feelings feel me. My heart is open. There is space enough for all of me.

*If it is important to avoid a sense of defeat,
it is equally important to avoid a sense of
guilt when progress or recovery may not
be possible.*
— Norman Cousins

We are all doing the best we can. If we could do any better, we would.

AIDS is still a mystery. We don't know why some of us get sick and some of us don't, why some of us get better and some of us don't. But we do know enough not to judge ourselves (or anyone else) if we aren't getting better. We do know not to judge ourselves for getting this disease in the first place. We do know that guilt and judgment contribute to disease, not recovery.

Instead of guilt, we can choose love. Instead of judgment, we can choose acceptance. When we choose love we remember that we are innocent children of a loving God and that none of this is punishment. It may just be our path this lifetime. Finally, when we choose acceptance, our sense of humor helps us detach a bit from our own drama; it protects us and keeps us from taking ourselves too seriously.

I choose love and acceptance. I choose not to take myself too seriously. I remember to step back now and then.

God speaks to all individuals through what
happens to them moment by moment.
— J. P. DeCaussade

When we listen to the messages given to us each
moment, we not only hear more clearly, we see
things differently too. We notice that the world is
quite beautiful.

In this moment, we know God is speaking to us.
We may sigh softly and smile. We know that we
are present with the great spirit of the universe. We
feel connected, safe, loved.

The trick is to pay attention. Often, our minds
wander ahead into the future or back to the past.
We know that we are not always here; we feel split
and disconnected. So we try to get our minds to
come back and live in the present with the rest of
us. Sometimes it takes a big crisis to get us to listen
and pay attention. For many of us, AIDS is that
crisis. It pulls us into the present so we can
hear our Higher Power speaking.

I take time to listen and meditate. I hear the voice of
God. I feel the presence of God. I see God all around
me. Where I am, there God is, speaking to me.

*When you meet anyone, remember it is
a holy encounter.*
— *A Course in Miracles*

Many of us are intent on avoiding people. In a crowd, we avoid touching others; we shift our eyes to avoid contact with strangers. Many of us have also spent years avoiding people we have unpleasant or unfinished business with.

The irony is, we all crave companionship. We want to feel part of a community. The Twelve Step program teaches us how to clear out all the unfinished business of our lives — how to let go of resentment and make amends. We learn how to face the past without shame or fear.

We learn to face the world head on, heart first, eyes open wide. We learn to meet people and be present with them. We learn to listen attentively and acknowledge their presence.

The more unfinished business we clear up the less distracted we are by fears and ghosts from the past, and the more present we can be with each person we meet. Being present and unafraid in the moment, we recognize God in other people.

*I will honor the divine in each person I meet today.
Each encounter will be holy.*

. . . the people who love you will appreciate knowing the truth. Give them that gift. And give yourself the gift of saying what's on your mind. Love yourself enough to tell the truth. TALK!
— Max Navarre, person with AIDS

There's no sense in trying to get through AIDS like a tough, macho movie hero. In real life, men and women who feel their feelings and are able to talk about them show true courage. Talking, like crying, screaming, or laughing, is an important way of expressing feelings. Sometimes, just talking can loosen us up enough to start energy moving through our whole body.

Talking to someone we trust is also a way we can discover what we are feeling. We often don't know until someone asks us, someone who we believe really wants to know. As we talk, feelings surface and we get in touch with ourselves.

And by being open with them, we give our friends, family, and lovers the opportunity to be open with us. What a lovely gift.

Today I will talk to someone about what's really on my mind and in my heart. I will go beyond the superficial. I will be intimate with at least one person today.

Each of you is a portion of God saying,
"I will create."

— *Emmanuel*

Each of us is a creative person. But sometimes we get blocked. Recovery and healing is really about removing blocks to our creativity; it's about being restored to our true place as spontaneous creators in this world.

As we go through life, we turn our experiences into beliefs. Some of those beliefs — low self-esteem, shame, guilt — block our creativity.

Our job is to uncover the beliefs that hold us back and change them. As we move those blocks aside, we clear a path for powerful energy to flow through us. The more blocks we dissolve in the light of understanding, the easier it is for the energy to flow.

As we become clear, open channels for the creative energy of the universe, we join with others to create a world of beauty and peace.

Show me the mistaken beliefs I hold that block the creative flow of energy through me. Help me dissolve them in the light of true understanding.

A guru might say that spiritual deepening involves a journey toward the unself-conscious living of life as it unfolds rather than toward a willful determination to make it happen.

— *John Fortunato*

What a relief to let go of our "willful determination to make it happen." For some of us, our first experience of giving up control happened when we admitted we were powerless over alcohol and other drugs. We didn't quit; we just gave up.

Letting go means we acknowledge that we don't have all the answers or even the best vision of how things ought to be for us. So things don't have to happen our way. We're willing to change course when the universe pushes us in a different direction.

Letting go doesn't mean we have no role in creating our lives. It means we remember to say at the end of our affirmations and visualizations "This or something better now manifests for me and for the good of all concerned. Not my will, but thine be done."

I am not responsible for making it happen. That I leave to God. I also trust that when I need to change direction, I'll get the message.

Men who are brave
And heroic
As you honor them to be,
Like them
I also
Consider myself to be.
    — *Ojibway War Song*
       Intepreted by Gerald Vizenor

All of us living with AIDS are brave. We are brave because we act even when we are afraid to act. One of the bravest things we do is reach out and ask for help; we ask another person into our lives.

We are brave when we admit that we can't do something, like taking on more responsibility, or walking another block, or continuing certain medical treatments.

Most importantly, we are brave every time we are honest about who we are. Throughout this epidemic, gay men have stood up in ever increasing numbers and demonstrated to the world what integrity means. Mothers and children with AIDS are showing the world what courage means. And there are families of people with AIDS who inspire us all.

I am an honest person. I speak the truth about who I am. I am brave, and I am proud of my life.

Each patient carries his own doctor inside him. They come to us not knowing that truth. We are at our best when we give the doctor who resides within each patient a chance to go to work.
— *Dr. Albert Schweitzer*

Living inside me is a great, knowing doctor, a healer. Am I giving this doctor a chance to work?

When I am afraid, in panic, I rush about looking for something to take, looking for someone to do something, always looking outside myself. When I act out of my fear, the doctor within can't help me because I'm not present. The doctor is in but the patient is out.

When I calm down, when I relax and breathe, when I center myself and bring my attention back to me, my healer can go to work.

Sometimes, slowing down is all we need to do. Other times, we may need to ask the healer in us for advice. We may feel awkward at first. Like any relationship, it takes time to build trust, but, after awhile, we'll both be very comfortable with each other.

Many times today, I will consult my internal doctor — the healer within. I will slow myself down and ask for Her advice.

Alcoholism (like all addictions) is not at base a search for utter sedation. It is a desire for the ecstasis, that 'standing out' from the landlocked lagoons of conformity, out onto the uncharted high seas where the only map is the star-set heavens.
— *Gerald Heard*

Alcohol and other drugs do "numb the pain" and many of us used them to do just that. But we also used them to try to reach beyond the mundane into the cosmic. After awhile, however, the transcendent experiences stopped happening, but we kept right on using.

Our addictions led us to a dead end. But our recovery is taking us down a path that has no end. We are learning that we don't need chemicals to experience the extraordinary. Living the spiritual life *is* living on the edge; it *is* dancing on the crest of ecstasy. We have boarded a star ship on a voyage of discovery in search of ourselves. We are searching, spiritual adventurers. And we are free to go as far as we want.

I am glad I am a seeker, a star searcher.

Most people are about as happy as they make their minds up to be.
— *Abraham Lincoln*

How we start our day has a lot to do with how it continues. No matter what attitude we wake up with, we can choose the attitude we wear for the rest of the day.

Before we get out of bed, we can run through an attitudinal checklist. It might look like this:

- Recall my dreams.
- Identify feelings present this morning.
- Accept them.
- Decide out loud what kind of day I want.
- Visualize having it. Experience how it feels.
- Open my heart and imagine golden white light streaming in, filling me with warmth and healing.

We can also make a list for the end of the day, taking inventory of the day and preparing for a wonderful night's rest.

Sometimes it seems that we don't have charge over very much. It's nice to remember that we always have charge over our attitude.

Every day I choose my attitude. God grant me the presence of mind to make a good choice.

So spend time every day listening to what
your muse is trying to tell you.
                                    — *Bartholomew*

We are all, each of us, incredibly creative people. If we think we aren't, we haven't been listening to our muse, that wonderful, playful, inner voice.

After years of being tuned out, how do we tune in? How do we become intimate with our muse? First, we have to commit to listening. Then we need to ask ourselves some personal questions: What makes me happy? What gives me delight? When do I feel deeply satisfied? When do I feel most in tune with myself? What am I afraid of? Am I afraid I won't be any good? By whose standards?

AIDS can be an excuse to isolate and feel sorry for ourselves and watch television. Or, it can be a great artistic awakener for all of us. What do we have to lose? In the face of this life-threatening disease, fear of not being as good as Picasso doesn't cut it.

God grant me the patience to listen to my muse and follow her suggestions. Help me remember that I am, by nature, creative and artistic.

Your body in illness is not your enemy
but your faithful friend...
Do heed its guidance.

— *Emmanuel*

"Well, good and faithful friend, what do you have to teach me today?"

Even in the midst of sickness, we can be delicate, polite, friendly, and respectful to ourselves. We can listen to what our body is trying to tell us.

Listening requires some relaxing. We won't be able to hear if we are uptight and scared. So we do whatever we do to relax. We breathe in, out, relax, and let go. We surrender to the moment, forget the past, stop worrying about the future, and breathe. We relax into the present and quietly listen to what our body is trying to tell us.

And even if the message isn't clear right away, we know that we have started a communication that is loving and respectful and that answers will come if we are patient.

I listen quietly and trust my body to tell me the truth.

A miracle can be thought of as a shift in perception that removes the fear and guilt that block our awareness of love's presence, which is our reality.
— *Gerald Jampolsky*

When a miracle happens, we experience peace, serenity, safety. We are, for a moment, aware of love's presence. We feel blessed, holy.

If we open to them, these miracles can happen many times each day. Being open to miracles may mean just sitting quietly in the afternoon sun. It may mean meditating, writing in a journal, or talking with a good friend.

Though being open to miracles may require lots of effort, it is important to remember that we are not responsible for making the miracle happen. We are only responsible for being willing to experience it.

We place ourselves in readiness. And then we ask: "Please remove all fear and guilt so that I may live in constant awareness of love's continual presence. Please remove all parts of me that block the light."

I am willing to let go of everything about me that casts a shadow over my awareness of love's constant presence. Please take them from me so I may live in the light.

. . .be open to all teachers and all teachings, and listen with your heart. With some you will feel you have no business. Others will pull you. Start to trust yourself.
— *Ram Dass*

A lot of what we call "personal growth" is simply replacing destructive habits with constructive habits. One new habit that can help heal our body, mind, and spirit is regular spiritual study.

For those of us uncomfortable with religion, we can open our mind to other forms of spirituality. If we keep our minds open and trust our hearts, we will be led along the right path.

Bookstores are full of resources for us. There are also lots of meetings, workshops, and lectures we can attend. If we follow our heart, and pay attention to our gut reaction, we will choose the books, workshops, guides, and teachers that are right for us.

I imagine myself walking in a heavenly garden where I joyfully pick flowers that brighten my soul. The flowers are my teachers, books, and guides. The bouquet I make is my own unique spiritual practice.

Zen Buddhists say that a finger is needed to point to the moon, but that we should not trouble ourselves with the finger once the moon is recognized.
— *Fritjof Capra*

The moon represents water and rules the oceans. As tides ebb and flow, the moon effortlessly shows her presence and power.

The moon is the symbol for our intuitive self. She holds sway over our emotions.

Every month the moon moves from full and bright to black and dark. Yet, even when we can't see her, her influence is felt. In the same way, even when we are not aware of our emotions they exist. They affect our health, our moods, our relationships, our energy.

The moon reminds us that just as water creates life in the desert or destroys coastlines, our emotions are powerful too. When we express our feelings, we nourish our souls. When we deny our feelings, we destroy ourselves.

The moon is our constant companion. She reminds us of our connection to all things seen and unseen. She reminds us of our need to be nurtured and to nurture.

I am one with the moon.

To link sexuality and intimacy is to link
sexuality with knowledge, with an opening
up of possibility rather than a closing down.
— David Mura

If we're mostly accustomed to anonymous or addictive sex, safer sex can be terrifying. Suddenly,
we're face to face with the reality of another living,
breathing, thinking, feeling human being.

In acknowledging these things in another person,
we acknowledge these things in ourselves. Intimate
sexuality not only opens up the possibility of getting to know someone else, it opens up the possibility of getting to know ourselves.

With intimacy, many things can happen: we're
not in control. With anonymity, only a limited
number of things can happen: we're in control.
Intimacy is risky, open. Anonymity is safe, closed.

AIDS is giving us the opportunity to move away
from anonymous, addictive, pornographic sex. The
old days are over. We cannot repeat the past. Now,
we can either hide out, or we can open up and risk
sexual intimacy.

---

*I choose to be intimate. I am willing to let go of my
need to control. I choose to open to the infinite possibilities of relationship.*

Feeling is a breath orgasm.
— *Joseph Kramer*

Feelings are intimately connected to breathing. When our moods change, our breathing changes. When we're calm and peaceful, our breathing is slow and regular. When we're frightened, our breathing is fast and irregular. When we're emotionally shut down, we may even forget to breathe.

Remembering to breathe keeps us conscious, living in the present moment, aware of our connection to the rest of life. Breathing connects us to every living being on earth. We're all breathing. And if we pay attention, we can feel all the world breathing together.

Conscious breathing can help us heal. One deep, lung-filling, satisfying breath can move us from feeling afraid to feeling loved. One exhale can create peace. Breathing is a miracle.

I am a conscious breather, a breathing healer. I am part of the living, breathing, pulsing, feeling, loving universe. I can feel it.

Perhaps one of the greatest rewards of meditation and prayer is the sense of belonging that comes to us.
— Bill Wilson

When we're sick, it's easy to feel separate from the world. While everyone else seems united in purpose, we feel like orphaned children: lost, frightened, and alone.

Prayer and meditation can become a loving, protective parent who holds us until we feel safe again. When we open our hearts in prayer and meditation, we realize that we are not alone; we remember that we are protected and included. We feel better the minute we move outside our fears and pray.

Happily, we can pray and meditate without knowing how. The key is to say, "I am willing." That's all. When we say, aloud or silently, "I am willing," we open our heart to love.

At any moment of the day, we can open ourselves in prayer and feel the peace of our Higher Power move through us. At any moment we can feel protected, watched over, cared for. At any moment we can know that we belong and that the world is safe.

I am willing. Hold me. Protect me. Watch over me. I am willing. Bathe me in light. Fill me with love.

It's so easy to lose our focus, to get lost in other people, external goals, and desires...we lose our connection to the universe inside ourselves. As long as we focus on the outside there will always be an empty, hungry, lost place inside that needs to be filled.

— *Shakti Gawain*

Most of us know what it's like to lose ourselves in a love affair, work, or sickness. We go months, even years without conscious contact with ourselves. We forget we exist apart from whatever it is we're lost in.

Then we remember, "Oh, I'm still here." For many of us, AIDS brings us back to remembering. It helps us focus on ourselves by teaching us what's important. It helps us stop running after external things. Because externals can't fill us up. They're like alcohol or other drugs: we keep wanting more.

What does fill us up is our attention, our love. When we bring our focus back to our feelings, our needs, our intuition, our goals, we get filled up. When we connect our little self to our God self, the emptiness disappears.

Help me find my way back from the land of the lost. Help me reconnect with my self, my inner knowing.

Nothing is predestined: The obstacles of your past can become the gateways that lead to new beginnings.

— *Ralph Blum*

It's easy to fall into the trap of believing that we are victims of circumstances, that real happiness is impossible in this lifetime because we are gay, or poor, or black, or addicted, or sick.

Even though we may have rebelled against them, some of those beliefs may still be lodged in our minds — unconscious judgments that say because of who we are, we can't have, do, or be what other people can have, do, or be.

The truth is this: those things that challenge us the most offer us the biggest opportunities. When we become friends with our difficulties they become our best teachers; they make us stronger. We realize that we are not victims of a world that happens to us. We choose for ourselves the perfect opportunities to learn and grow and become.

We realize that because of who we are, real happiness is possible this lifetime.

I let go of all limiting beliefs and allow fate to unfold moment by moment. What I thought were obstacles I now see are doorways to new possibilities and new beginnings.

The basic teaching of Buddhism is the teaching of transiency, or change. That everything changes is the basic truth for each existence.

— *Shunryu Suzuki*

Much of the anxiety in our lives is caused by our struggle to keep from changing. Much of our fear, including our fear of dying, is really fear of change, fear that we will disappear, lose ourselves in the cosmic mist.

Fighting against a law of nature is bound to create anxiety. And the law that everything changes is nature's most basic law. Even who we are changes. Our bodies change, our circumstances change, and the way we look at the world changes.

When we accept and move with the laws of nature we are released from anxiety and we are free to express our true, unique self. We don't lose ourselves; we find ourselves. Letting go of our resistance to what we cannot resist, frees up energy for healing, for play, for happiness, and for loving.

I lovingly let go of my attachment to my present self and fearlessly move into the flow of my becoming.

There is no such thing as a problem without a gift for you in its hand. You seek problems because you need their gifts.
— A Course in Miracles

Because of AIDS, many of us are healing our relationships, including those with our family, something we thought might never be possible.

Because of AIDS, some of us are learning to treat ourselves with kindness and generosity. We love and accept ourselves just as we are. We are taking good care of ourselves.

Because of AIDS, some of us are growing spiritually. We have a new relationship with God, however we understand God.

Because of AIDS, we are becoming the kind of people we always wanted to be — always deep down believed we were. We are discovering that we are kind, loving, empowered, confident, spiritual, creative, and friendly.

AIDS is a tragedy only when we don't see the gifts it brings.

I am grateful for the gifts my problems bring to me. Help me always be aware of what they are.

. . .the reward of patience is patience.
— *St. Augustine*

If we are patient, we will have patience. Patience breeds patience. It allows us to move with the flow of nature, to breathe in time to the breathing of the earth. Patience is the name for the rhythm of harmony.

After so many years of wanting things to happen "my way," finally letting go of our demands is a great relief.

Patience works hand in hand with trust. When we trust that events are unfolding according to plan, we can relax and be patient. When we trust in God's will for us, we don't worry about working our will. When we trust all that happens will be exactly right for us, we are free to live in the moment.

Patience is healing. When we are patient with ourselves, with our process, with our recovery, with our body, we are able to let go of disease-causing stress. We can relax into our healing.

I live in this moment. I am patient with myself. I trust the universe. I am free.

Depression follows panic... and depression is an intensifying cause of illness. The mood of the patient, therefore, is hardly of less concern to the physician than the disease he is called upon to treat.
— Norman Cousins

There is too much panic around AIDS. We panic when we find out we have HIV antibodies. We panic because friends test positive. We panic when blood tests come back. But panic causes depression that contributes to illness. We need to try to replace panic with confidence. Hope follows confidence, and hope contributes to health. Hope expects health.

It's easier to choose confidence and avoid panic if we listen more to positive, hopeful people and less to negative, fearful people. If our doctors and friends are giving us panic-causing messages, we need to ask them to change their attitude, or we need to find new doctors and new friends.

Our healers and the people who love and support us can help us fight panic and depression. Together, we can choose confidence and hope.

There is no reason to panic. I am held in the hand of God. I am confident and hopeful. I surround myself with confident, hopeful people.

It is essential to recognize that the needs being met through the illness are fully legitimate *and* deserve *to be met. The body is demanding attention in the only way it knows how.*
— Carl and Stephanie Simonton

When we get sick, one of the most important questions we can ask is, "What needs am I getting met through this illness?" Maybe we're getting attention; we need and deserve lots of attention. Maybe we're getting love and affection; we need and deserve unlimited love and affection. Maybe we're emotionally, physically, or spiritually exhausted and we need a rest. We all need and deserve time off.

Or, maybe we're becoming aware of how painful our lives have been; we're saying that we don't want to keep on as we've been going.

Whatever we come up with is okay. There is no shame in having needs; it's part of being human. The point is to get those human needs met through being well.

I bless my body for helping me learn more about myself. I accept myself and my human needs. I commit to giving all my needs direct and kind attention.

To a distant land
He is going
My lover
Soon
He will come again.
— *Ojibway Love Song*
Interpreted by Gerald Vizenor

In almost all stories about heroes, the hero goes away and comes back. From the King Arthur legend to Star Wars, heroes leave home, go on adventures, face danger, and, finally, return home transformed. Like Luke Skywalker, they find the source for the strength and courage they need within themselves. They bring back the message that what we thought we needed from "out there," we already have "in here."

We are all heroes, called to leave home, face adventures, learn lessons, and return, wiser, more aware of who we are. For us, AIDS is part of our adventure. Through this trial we are becoming more confident and empowered. We are discovering that the force goes with us, that the source of power is in the heart of the hero.

I am on a great adventure of transformation. The force is with me.

No God of loving compassion
would ever inflict upon anyone . . .
any illness at all.

— *Emmanuel*

Those who believe AIDS is God's punishment are projecting their own guilt. We have no control over what they believe, but we can beware of our own self-destructive guilt. We may not always be aware of guilt. But where guilt is, fear isn't far behind. So, whenever we feel fear, we might also be on the lookout for guilt.

Then, we need to remember to choose love instead of fear, forgiveness instead of guilt and blame.

When we do, AIDS becomes our gift, our opportunity to learn and grow and become, each day, more aware of our own godliness. AIDS becomes our chance to draw closer into loving community. It also becomes our opportunity to expand outward to include more people in our world of love, understanding, and acceptance.

God of loving compassion, kind spirit of the universe, release me from the prison of guilt. Allow me to see myself through your eyes — innocent and pure. Help me project only love and safety.

September

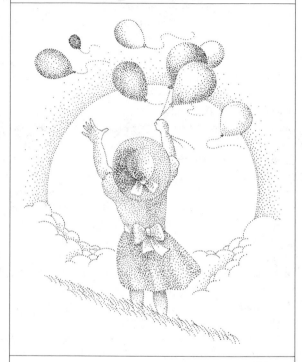

Today I celebrate the sun's birthday. I celebrate my rebirth. Break out the balloons.

*To live with shame is to feel alienated and
defeated, never quite good enough to belong. And secretly we feel to blame. Shame
is without parallel a sickness of the soul.*
— *Gershen Kaufman*

Most of us know what shame feels like. It's a pain
that comes from believing we aren't good enough.
And it persists as long as we have no name for it,
or have no answers to its accusations.

Once we recognize it and name it we can see what
a horrible mistake was made. We *do* qualify. We
are good enough. Now that we can name it and
talk to other people about it, we're able to answer
shame's accusations with positive affirmations.
We're able to look back and see that people have
always accepted us just the way we are, as perfectly
good, imperfect human beings.

As we begin to heal from the soul sickness called
shame, we'll need reassurance and acceptance. Every
day, we need to tell ourselves that we are loved and
we belong.

*The antidote to shame's poison is love. I am filled
with love.*

We are living in a very exciting and power-
ful time. On the deepest level of conscious-
ness, a radical spiritual transformation is
taking place.

— *Shakti Gawain*

Something really profound is happening on our
planet. Spiritually speaking, we are waking up. We
are remembering who we are.

This spiritual awakening is reflected in those of
us dealing with AIDS. Because of AIDS, we are
growing spiritually. We are letting go of a lot of the
external things we thought were important, and we
are discovering who we really are. We are giving
up the desperate scramble for things, no longer
basing our worth on what we have or how we look.
We are each coming to in our own way, on our own
schedule. As we look around us, we see that we
are not alone. We are part of a ground swell, a
revolution, a transformation of humanity.

Today I will focus my attention on the spiritual trans-
formation that is happening to me, to my friends, and
to our planet.

This is perhaps the most difficult of the balancing acts we come to learn: to trust the pain as well as the light, to allow the grief to penetrate as it will while keeping open to the perfection of the universe.
— *Stephen Levine*

No matter how great our faith, when someone we love dies, we grieve. Even if we truly believe death is an illusion, there is still penetrating, demanding grief. Even if we truly believe lives are unfolding as they should, we still cry out in our suffering.

Within each of us there is an ocean of grief, a seemingly inexhaustible well of sadness and loss. Every time we grieve, we tap into that ancient pool of pain, we open our hearts and become vulnerable. For some reason, we sometimes also feel connected, joined with everything that ever was and ever will be. Our grief leads us through the darkness back into the light. In our despair we find new belief.

Even when my grief tests my faith, I am not far from the light. I trust even when I don't understand.

My behavior was not what needed to be changed. It was my feelings about myself that needed to be changed. My behavior was just an outward reflection of what was going on inside.
— *George Melton, person recovering from AIDS*

Most of us know what it's like to struggle with problem-causing behaviors. It's very frustrating. Sheer willpower doesn't work against drinking, drug abuse, smoking, or overeating because compulsive behavior is a symptom, an external sign of something internal.

If we're abusing ourselves on the outside, we've probably got an abusive voice raging at us on the inside, telling us that because of who we are, we don't deserve love and kindness.

The first thing we need to do is change the internal message. We need to record messages of total love and acceptance. We need to hear voices that tell us we are wonderful, creative, and deserving of all good things.

My behavior flows from my beliefs. I believe that I am safe and secure. I believe that I am a miraculous example of love in motion.

Does this path have a heart?
— Carlos Castenada

Whenever we need to decide on a way to go, we can ask, "Does this path have a heart? Is love present? Does this path make me feel serene and hopeful? Is this the path to peace? What are the people on this path like?"

Whether we're choosing a spiritual direction, choosing a career, joining an organization, or making a treatment decision, we can always let our heart guide us. Heart recognizes heart. To learn if a path has heart we need to listen to our own.

Breathing deeply, in and out, sinking our roots deep into the center of the earth, we bring our attention to our heart, and listen. Quietly, the answers come, the feelings surface.

As we make decisions based on our heart's knowing, we realize that we need never again walk on a path that doesn't have heart.

I am on a path with heart. Every step I make brings me closer to the light. I walk in the presence of love. I am at peace.

The instant that the Self
releases from the human body,
there is Light, there is peace,
there is freedom, there is Home.
— *Emmanuel*

When we forget who we really are and think of ourselves as just bodies with personalities, we naturally become afraid, especially of death.

But when we remember that we are much more than our bodies, when we remember our spirit essence, we realize that our body is just a temporary form, a form perfectly suited to learn what we need to learn on earth. When we identify with our spirit, we remember our connection to all spirit, to the moving energy and light that is the essence of all people and living things.

We realize that we are constantly changing and moving energy — eternal, always becoming. Death is not an ending; it is part of becoming, part of an unbroken continuation.

I am more than my body. I am spirit, a being of light, a creator with God of this ever-changing and expanding universe. I am becoming.

Sometimes
I go about pitying
Myself,
While I am carried
By the wind
Across the sky.
  — *Ojibway Dream Song*
   Interpreted by Gerald Vizenor

When we forget who we are, we identify with our problems: I am AIDS, I am sickness. When we forget who we are, we run the risk of sinking into the swamp of self-pity.

One good way to remember who we are is to take a walk outside. (If we can't actually go outside, we can imagine being outside.) While walking, under the sky, on the earth, little things like the wind pushing the clouds can remind us of who we are. We remember that we are old souls. We share the rhythms of the sun and the moon, oceans and deserts — not hospitals or clinics, offices or factories. Our heartbeat is the ancient drumbeat, the pulse of nature.

Even if I forget who I am, I am still carried by the wind across the sky. I am supported by the earth and cared for by the Creator God.

Follow your bliss. Find where it is and don't be afraid to follow it.
— *Joseph Campbell*

Whatever we dream of doing, we must try to do it. And if we don't know what our dreams are, we must discover them.

Long ago, many of us were shamed with words like, "You can't." "You won't." "How dare you?" "Who do you think you are?" So, to protect our dreams, we hid them, buried them deep inside. We didn't want them discounted, tarnished, ridiculed.

It's time to go find them, dig them up, resurrect them. For some of us, this may be simple. Others of us may have to be more creative; we may have to do some childlike dreaming again.

If we take our resurrected dreams and combine them with what gives us pleasure now, we will find our bliss. Then it's up to us to follow it. No more doubting or disbelieving; it's time to act and trust that when we are being true to ourselves, the universe supports us in every way.

I uncover the secret dreams of my heart, hold them up to the light, and follow them wherever they lead.

We see the world piece by piece, as the sun, the moon, the animal, the tree; but the Whole, of which these are shining parts, is the Soul.

— *Ralph Waldo Emerson*

It's no wonder that sometimes we feel fragmented and disjointed. The world looks like it's divided into billions of pieces, all separate and distinct. What is the force that unites all the parts and keeps everything from colliding in random motion? Is there a Whole?

Emerson called it the Soul. Others call it the Life Force, Brahman, the movement of energy, Higher Power, God.

If we imagine the Whole is the Soul and we acknowledge that each of us also has a Soul, or is a Soul, then, we have outlined the great paradox, the mystery of the universe: All that is out there, everything on earth and in the heavens, is also part of us. We reflect the majesty of all the pieces and all the pieces are a reflection of us. To know the whole, the unifying thing itself, we must turn to our own Soul and get to know the God within.

My life is one piece, a Whole, just as the world is one piece, a Whole. Contained in my Soul is all the mystery and magic of the universe.

Your misery comes when you tighten up, when you do not allow your agony to move. . . . The more you believe you should be isolated when you are in a bad mood, the worse you feel.

— *Bartholomew*

Many of us feel like we always have to be the perfect host or hostess even when we're lying flat on our backs in the hospital. There we lay, irritated, afraid, angry, and still smiling sweetly.

It comes from old lessons we learned about how good boys and girls behave. Boys don't cry and girls don't get mad. So here we are, facing a life-threatening illness, with simplistic ideas about how we should behave. Boys do cry and girls do get mad. If we let ourselves cry, scream, and storm about, we open up the paths for our pain to move.

Real freedom comes when we openly and honestly express ourselves to the people around us. We free ourselves and show others in our lives how to be real, present, alive, and honest.

I find the tight places in my body where I am holding on, and I release and let go. I do not try to protect people from how I feel. I am honest and offer my feelings as gifts.

...the journey begins by quieting one's insides, making room, leaving time to hear and to notice...the practice of spiritual growth has as its core the practice of silence.

— John Fortunato

The messages are coming through. The guidance we need is here. All we need to know is available to us. We aren't missing any pieces. We do need to be quiet, though, because messages come through most clearly in silence.

Most spiritual practices are designed to make us better listeners. They help remove static and ego interference. They help us sit in silence. The important thing to remember is that we don't need to wait until we're perfect receivers before we tune in. We only need to be willing to listen.

And the messages we receive today will guide us further down the path of spiritual growth.

It's a simple, two-step process: calm the mind and listen.

I sit still. I breathe in spirit and exhale all tension, noise, and discomfort. One by one, from the top of my head to the bottoms of my feet, I relax my muscles. I am like a tree, rooted in the earth, reaching toward the sky, breathing, listening.

The more willing you are to surrender to the energy within you, the more power can flow through you.

— *Shakti Gawain*

For some of us, the problem with spirituality is that it usually gets around to God. And for us, God has always been a distant, angry, hard-to-approach authority figure. Yet, the root of the word spirituality is spirit, not God. We don't have to believe in God to claim our own spirituality.

And spirit isn't something set apart from us. It's inside us. It surrounds us. It's the energy moving through the trees, mountains, rivers, and other people. When we accept that this energy is moving through us, we understand that we are, by nature, connected and part of the whole.

When we stop fighting our spiritual nature and surrender to it, we open the flood gates and allow more energy to flow through us; we become empowered. We are given the strength to do what we couldn't before. As we let go, we are given the strength to more easily and effortlessly express our true, unique selves.

I willingly surrender to a Higher Power, the energy moving inside me.

> *...conquest of panic is an essential part of any recovery program from a serious disease.*
>
> — *Norman Cousins*

Sometimes it seems like the gay community is in the grip of an AIDS panic. We're in a heightened state of anxiety from which there seems little relief, except to finally get diagnosed.

We need to diffuse this panic. We need to acknowledge our fear, apprehension, and panic. Then we need to give ourselves our fullest, kindest, most gentle, loving, and accepting attention.

We must also support each other in being well. We know we can be supportive when we're sick. We need to be even more encouraging to each other about recovery and health.

And finally, we can each live today, just today, moment by moment. Panic is future-oriented. When we focus on the present, we connect to powerful, healing, health-sustaining energy.

I accept all my feelings and surround them in love. I live in the present: calm, connected, peaceful, and unafraid.

I'm beginning to see my cancer as something that the Soul-me planned to have happen because the Wingate-me needed it for his growth.
— Wingate Paine

Whether it's cancer, AIDS, or a broken arm, the question is always, why? Why now? Why this? What am I supposed to learn? No one can answer these questions for us. Others can tell us about their journey, but they can't tell us our truth.

We have to find that out for ourselves. It's our adventure. Sitting quietly, we listen for our truth; we listen to find out why AIDS, why us. Along the way, we may find clues in books, workshops, or support groups.

It is also possible that while living our lives, answers will come to us in lightning bolts of inspiration. Suddenly, we know. We see the reason in the smile of a friend, or a feeling moves through our body — and we know.

The answers come if we ask the questions and are open to hearing the reply.

I am willing to learn the lessons of my life's experiences. I open to understanding my soul's wisdom.

*You wouldn't believe the number of people
diagnosed with AIDS who still haven't told
their families.*
— Archie, person with AIDS

Hiding who we are from our families causes us
stress. We have to be on stage, dishonest, pretend-
ing, tense.

Most of us know what it's like to hide something
important about ourselves from our family. Maybe
we haven't told our families about our AIDS diagnosis, or about being gay, or about our drug use,
or about our recovery.

AIDS is teaching us that there is no time like now
to begin healing our family relationships, which
means we start communicating. We come out of
whatever closet we're hiding in and get honest. As
we do, we remember we're not responsible for our
parents' reactions; we can't control how they
respond. What we can do is start the process of
forgiving ourselves and our parents, completely.

---

*Today I pray for the courage to be current and honest
about who I am in the presence of my family. Help
me heal all my relationships, especially my relationship with my parents.*

If I had my life to live over, I would start barefoot earlier in the spring and stay that way later in the fall. I would go to more dances. I would ride more merry-go-rounds. I would pick more daisies.
— Nadine Stair

We can't relive our lives, but we can choose today to live the way we have always wanted to live. Whether we are conscious of it or not, each day we make a choice. We choose to continue as we've been going or we choose to change.

Today we can decide to live like the kind of grown-up person who hops on merry-go-rounds, picks daisies, and dances. We can lay in the grass and watch ants work. We can choose to live today with no regrets about the past. After all, our past brought us to this marvelous place, this moment of creation, this totally new day.

What will we be like today? Will we be sullen and worried, or bright and positive? Will we be spontaneous, active, and creative? It's our choice.

Today I will live my life the way I would live it if I had it to live over.

*There are trees that seem to die at the end
of autumn. There are also the evergreens.*
— *Gilbert Maxwell*

Among us are people who are like evergreens.
They keep hope alive in themselves and radiate
hope for the rest of us.

They stand tall, sometimes alone, sometimes with
others. They tell us that we have choices. They
challenge us to be powerful creators of our lives.
They refuse to be victims.

They build organizations, speak to the press, and
sometimes disappear for a while in order to grow
strong again. Most of all, they teach us that AIDS
is a fightable disease and that we are powerful
people. They teach us how to love and accept ourselves, that this is our strongest defense. They teach
us how to be survivors, evergreens.

---

*I honor the memories of those who are gone, and I
bless and honor the presence of those among us who
stand like evergreens.*

I've learned more in the last year about myself than I had in the previous eighteen. I spent those eighteen years very numb. I tried to numb myself out, to build walls around myself with work, with alcohol, with bad relationships.
    — *Mark Christopherson, person with AIDS*

We may have given up the obvious ways to stay numb: alcohol, other drugs, sex, compulsive eating. But many of us still fall into the "always on the move" trap. We keep moving; we never slow down.

Sometimes it takes getting sick to slow us down long enough to come back to life, to regain that tingling that reminds us we are still alive, here, present in this moment.

We don't have to wait until we get sick. We can take time each day to get to know ourselves. We can talk about what's happening and how we feel. Like good friends who haven't seen each other for a long, long time, we can spend time in delicious conversation.

I happily spend time with myself. I'm like a reunion inside; all parts of me are getting reacquainted. I realize that I love this complicated person I call me.

*Often inside the addict is a boy who did
not learn the word pleasure.... When sex
entered the boy's life there was no word
for pleasure to name it. It was sin, it
was work.*

— David Mura

Pleasure and Sex. A happy combination. Yes?
Well, how does it feel to sit for a moment with those
two words together?

For many of us it doesn't feel happy. It feels sad.
Because, as children, someone forgot to teach us
about pleasure. So we attached other words to sex:
guilt and shame.

For many of us, our first experiences of sexual
pleasure were linked with deep shame, secrecy,
abuse. We became locked in a sexual nightmare
based on guilt, compulsion, and obsession.

It's time to learn the word *pleasure*. It's time to
let go of guilt — all of it. It's time to claim our sexuality, to take our sexuality out of the dark and put
it into a big, open, sunlit space. Ironically, it may
be that the honesty and openness needed to practice safer sex will help us learn to enjoy our sexuality, to finally combine pleasure with sex.

*I easily and effortlessly balance work and pleasure. I
love my pleasure-seeking, sexual self.*

*I sin if I submit to the indignities that are
hurled at me. I am a guardian of the divine
dignity and it is my duty to defend it.*
— *Chief Albert Luthuli*

Many of us are learning to feel empowered and
to express our newfound self-esteem. In the past,
we were more likely to feel shameful and unworthy
than proud and dignified. When we did act assured,
we were often trying to cover up our true insecurity.

Somewhere along the line, probably when we
were young, we decided against ourselves. Now
we can change and decide for ourselves. Because
the truth is we are very special people. We are how
God is expressed on earth.

So when we stand up for ourselves and say it's
not okay to treat me badly, we become filled with
more spirit. When we recognize and reject insult
coming at us or at our brothers and sisters, we make
ourselves stronger.

*I honor and respect myself. I honor and respect every-
one I meet. I expect and receive honor in return.*

Those who die relearn, or remember, the secrets of Life that they forgot at birth.
— *Elizabeth Johnson*

We are all in the process of remembering what we forgot at birth. Each time we are transformed through change, each time we let go of an old behavior, habit, or attitude, our old self dies, and we remember more.

It is the process of spiritual awakening. As we come to, we remember that we are more than bodies; we are also spirit and soul. Our soul is ancient. It knows that we have always had a deep spiritual kinship with everyone. Our soul knows the secrets of life.

As we awaken, we learn to trust this process of death and rebirth that transforms us. As we awaken, it becomes easier to accept dying as just another part of that continual process — another transformation from which we emerge again, reborn, remembering who we are, remembering the secrets of life.

I am open to the process of transformation. Help me remember who I am. Teach me again the secrets of life.

Is this not life's purpose —
to know that you belong,
that you are safe and eternal,
to know that in your spirit reality
you are already one with God?
                              — *Emmanuel*

Most of us know what it's like to feel we don't belong, to feel separate and alienated from other people and from God. Because AIDS forces us to look for help from other people, it can teach us that we do belong. As we open our heart and allow ourselves to receive loving support from other people, we feel connected, one with others, maybe for the first time.

And because AIDS is life-threatening, it makes us think about who we are beyond our body. It makes us aware of our spirit.

So if we're feeling alienated and unsafe, we can reach out and ask for help. We can pick up the phone or go to a support group. And we can pray for awareness of our connection to the world of spirit. Miracles of change are set in motion through a simple prayer. Prayer is a powerful form of reaching out. Prayer reminds us that all we have to do is ask.

God help me feel safe, secure, and one with the universe.

Forgiveness means letting go of the past.
— Gerald Jampolsky

We all know how guilt and blame keep us constantly ashamed of our past and worried about our future. We know how heavy resentments can become when we carry them around day after day. Forgiveness lightens our load and lets us live in the present.

The process of forgiveness may have to include making amends for past behavior. It may mean owning up to things we'd just as soon deny. It may even bring us face to face with our anger and our sadness.

Whatever we have to do, we don't have to do it all at once. All we need to be is willing to let go of the past. If we aren't ready today, we only need to be willing to be ready sometime in the future.

We need only be willing to do whatever is necessary to finally look back at our past and smile, knowing that that's what it took to bring us to this moment.

God grant me willingness to forgive myself and everyone else. Help me let go of the past.

*The intuitive hunch is always there. What
I started to do was live my life following
those hunches.*
— Will Garcia, person recovering
from AIDS

The intuitive hunch may always be there but we
aren't always listening. Even when we do hear it,
deciding to follow our intuition instead of the course
laid out by our rational mind usually takes a running leap of faith.

Because it's hard to trust, even though we all know
from our own experiences that when we follow our
hunches, things usually turn out for the best.

The problem is, when we try to follow our
hunches, our ego rebels. We're placing mind at the
service of heart and our ego doesn't like that one
bit. But sooner or later, ego gets over himself and
realizes that mind is much happier carrying out the
wishes of heart.

Then, we worry less and trust more. We know
we are following our higher good. We also become
open to wonderful surprises. We begin to see
that as we give up trying to control everything,
magic happens.

I open my heart and follow my hunches.

Scorpio is the eternal question tearing at all roots under autumnal skies. Will it be death; will it be rebirth?
— Dane Rudhyar

Autumn is a good time to meditate on the deep mysteries of death and transformation. In autumn, the world goes underground. Leaves fall off trees. Days get shorter. Plants turn brown. The world gets dark in preparation for the rebirth of light.

How do we become reborn unless we also allow parts of ourselves to die and fall away? Old ideas, old behaviors, limitations we clinged to in the past can now be shed. The person we are dies. We become another person, someone who more closely resembles what we want to become.

For this magical transformation, only willingness is needed. Courage will be supplied. We need only be willing to risk being naked for a time, without our props and familiar routines. We need only be willing to risk finding out more about ourselves.

I willingly surrender. I let go of all old behaviors and beliefs that no longer serve me. I am transformed.

*We can always perceive others as either
extending love or giving a call for help.*
— A principle of the Center for
Attitudinal Healing

Let's face it, most of our anxiety comes from our contact with other people. We have to deal with lovers, spouses, co-workers, doctors, nurses, bad drivers, and neighbors with barking dogs. And on any one day some of them are disappointing us, behaving badly, being disagreeable, or ignoring us.

No wonder we feel threatened. Our safety is at stake. So we use up a lot of energy being anxious. Sometimes it seems like we don't have any other choice, but we really do. We can choose to worry, or we can choose to see other people as either extending love or calling for help. When we choose not to worry, we have a lot of energy available to pour into our own lives, and more energy to extend love to everyone we meet.

*I choose my attitude. Today I choose to perceive everyone
I meet as either extending love or asking for help.*

At first you will think of your sadhana
*[spiritual practice] as a limited part of your
life. In time you will come to realize that
everything you do is part of your* sadhana.
— *Ram Dass*

Many of us began our spiritual path because we
didn't have a choice. Alcohol or other drugs had
us licked. We were willing to try anything. AIDS
is like that too. It's something we can't handle
alone. So we join forces with a Power greater
than ourselves.

We start our practice. We may start with a book,
a group, a spiritual advisor, or we may simply start
to pray. Slowly we begin to realize that everything
we do — our work, our play, our sexual activity
— is part of our spiritual practice. Everything can
lead us to a closer relationship to our spiritual self.

Whether we're in a cathedral, a Zen center, or a
hospital waiting room, we can practice our sadhana.

---

*Everything I do is a sacred ritual. Every moment is
a communion. I feel the healing presence of spirit all
around me. Spirit enters my body and bathes me in
light and love.*

No one dies unless the life force of that person agrees to leave the planet.
— Elizabeth Johnson

Sometimes we feel guilty when someone we love dies. We think we could have or should have done more to show that person our love. But, dying is a very personal thing. Someone else's death is not about us. (That's one reason why we feel such painful separation and loneliness when someone we love leaves his or her body. It is clearly their trip.)

And at least on some deep level of understanding, that person agreed to leave. If our soul is not ready, we will not die, regardless of our condition. If our soul is ready, we will leave, regardless of what anybody else does or doesn't do. So, there is no reason to blame ourselves or blame other people. Dying is very personal.

We only need to say good-bye, trusting that the person is on a new adventure, just as we continue our great adventure, incarnate on planet earth.

I trust that dying, like all parts of my spiritual journey, will happen at exactly the right time. And so, I do not worry about myself, and I do not worry about my friends.

His dog up and died,
Up and died.
After twenty years,
He still grieved.
— *"Mr. Bojangles" by Jerry Jeff Walker*

Over time, grief's pain becomes less intense. We return to our routines. We laugh and smile more easily. Yet sometimes, for no apparent reason, we touch it. Talking to friends or just daydreaming, our eyes well up with tears. Sometimes we know who the tears are for, sometimes we don't.

AIDS requires that we grieve. It can give us a chance to grieve deeply. It can give us an opening to all our sadness, all our unexpressed grief, and unacknowledged loss. AIDS can give us access to the place that holds vast feeling, our reservoir of tears. Once there, we don't need to understand whether our grief is current or old or who it's for. The important thing is to have it, to cry when we feel like crying, to be sad when we're sad, and to talk about our losses.

I've had lots of losses, lots of accumulated grief. Grief will visit me for the rest of my life. I am grateful to be able to feel its cleansing presence.

Believing that I could survive is probably the precondition necessary for my survival. Unlike many other people with AIDS who considered themselves "ticking time bombs," my worldview admitted from the first at least the possibility of recovery.
— Michael Callen, person with AIDS

Belief that we can survive, from AIDS or any other life-threatening illness, makes recovery possible. But because what we believe is often hidden from us, we need to look for it. Sitting quietly, breathing deeply, we need to ask ourselves, "What do I believe about AIDS? What do I believe about me?"

If we feel hopeless and lean toward the "ticking time bomb" theory of AIDS, we will want to make some changes, which isn't so hard. Beliefs are just ideas we chose to accept. There are other ideas about AIDS and we can decide to accept them.

If each day we affirm the idea that we can survive, thrive, recover and be happy, our affirmations will become beliefs, our beliefs will become images, and our images will help create our world.

I believe that it is possible to survive. I believe that it is possible to recover from AIDS. Every day in every way, I grow stronger, healthier, more alive.

October

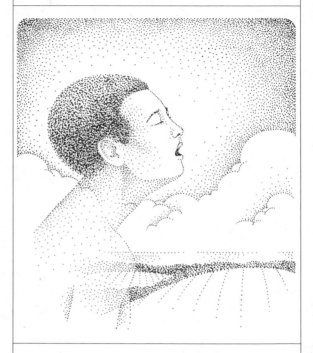

I vibrate in harmony. I joyfully reclaim lost parts of myself that were once mute but now sing in chorus with the rest of me.

Were it possible for us to see further than our knowledge reaches, perhaps we would endure our sadnesses with greater confidence than our joys. For they are moments when something new has entered into us, something unknown; our feelings grow mute in shy perplexity, everything in us withdraws, a stillness comes, and the new, which no one knows, stands in the midst of it and is silent.

— *Rainer Maria Rilke*

In moments of sadness, the seeds of new growth are planted. Sometimes we cry because we know that the person we are will soon disappear, transformed into someone else, someone closer to who we really are.

In these moments, we realize that the world is more mysterious and wonderful than anyone has ever been able to explain. Faced with this truth, tears come to our eyes, not unhappy tears, tears of transformation.

In sadness, I sit alone in silence. I welcome the new and let go of the old. I welcome the transformation. I am grateful for my tears.

The body is the reactor.
It vibrates to stress
and is an outward manifestation
of inner turmoil.

— *Emmanuel*

Life is stressful. How we respond — mentally, emotionally, spiritually — affects our bodies. Our bodies are like tuning forks. They carry the pitch, but are not the source of the vibration. How we translate life's challenges into our emotions and how we express those emotions determines whether we vibrate freely and easily or whether we block up.

That's why we try to go with the flow, to let go and let God. We try to live one day at a time. That's also why we practice forgiveness. When we forgive ourselves and others and let go of guilt and blame, we dislodge old emotions, old stress stuck somewhere in our body. We experience our denied emotions, so they don't have to disguise themselves as sickness or depression.

I vibrate in harmony. I joyfully reclaim parts of me that were once mute but now sing in chorus with the rest of me.

What is to worship an image? It is to pray for a gift you will never receive.
— David Mura

When the real world is so incredibly abundant, how painful and sad to be obsessed with the unreal images portrayed in pornography and advertising, images that tell us how we should look and what we should want. These images promote self-hate and hopelessness.

With awareness, we can pull away from the lost world of craving images. Being aware of where we focus our attention and where our minds wander makes us honest. If we are aware, we can bring our attention back to ourselves, to this moment, to reality. We can step out of the violent world where images of what we're supposed to be continually bash against the reality of who we truly are.

Instead, we step into a peaceful world of loving self-acceptance and honest acknowledgment of who we are, right now. Then, in peace, our hearts can open and receive real blessings from an abundant universe.

I am aware of my thoughts, this moment. In peace, I accept myself exactly as I am. With humility, I open my heart to receive, without exception, all the gifts the universe has to give.

I exist as I am, that is enough,
If no other in the world be aware I
  sit content,
And if each and all be aware I sit content.
— *Walt Whitman*

When we're feeling low and we're afraid we aren't good enough, we can practice self-affirmation — active, positive self-acceptance. We can affirm, "I am what I am."

Daily doses of "I am what I am" therapy is an antidote to the poison of perfectionism. Many of us grew up believing that approval depended on what we did. And we could never do enough, good enough. So today, we still worry that we aren't acceptable, that we are never finished, presentable, good enough.

As we practice self-acceptance, we let go of that old anxiety. The more we tell ourselves we are fine just the way we are, the less worry we have about what others think. We become less self-conscious, more relaxed. We discover that people like us just the way we are.

All day long, whether I am conscious of it or not, I will receive positive messages that say, "I am perfect today in every way."

We sometimes congratulate ourselves at the moment of waking from a troubled dream: it may be so the moment after death.

— *Nathaniel Hawthorne*

It's a good idea to occasionally think about dying, to think about how it will be and what we might expect. Trying to understand death can take away our fear of it, just as shining a light on a shadow makes it disappear.

Many people who have had near death experiences, who have "died" and come back, tell about bright lights at the end of tunnels, profound peace and security, and about being met and guided by friendly beings of light. They return to life, no longer afraid of death, no longer afraid of life either.

After we think about dying, after we sit quietly and uncover what we feel and know about death, we might also want to think about living. What can we do to make our living less troubled, more happy? Where is fear holding us back from living as fully as we can?

As I honestly face the possibility of my death, I lose my fear of dying and become more fearless in my living.

*I do not know whether I was then a man
dreaming I was a butterfly, or whether I
am now a butterfly dreaming I am a man.*
— *Chuang Tzu*

We are taught to assume that our rational mind
knows what is true and real and that our dreams
and fantasies are unreal. How do we know?

Using our rational mind we change the world,
chopping down forests, building houses, diagnos-
ing illnesses, and prescribing treatments. We do
many things that prove our rational mind is in touch
with reality.

Yet, our dreaming, intuitive mind also helps us
build our world. We create soaring skyscrapers, ele-
gant bridges, and inspiring music because we were
able to dream them. We transform lives and cure
"incurable" diseases with imagination and believing.

Everywhere we turn we prove that our dreaming, intuitive mind is as true, real, and important
as our rational mind. Both contribute to who we
are. We stay in balance by nurturing both.

---

*I love my practical, rational self and I love my intui-
tive, imaginative self. I honor and respect them both.*

Simply sit quietly, take a few deep breaths,
and focus your awareness within — to the
wise being within you who is in touch with
the wisdom of the universe.
             — Shakti Gawain

Often, when we're anxious, afraid, or angry, we feel trapped in our mood. It feels like there's no way out. Tension builds in us, and we become even more anxious.

There is a way out. We always have a choice. If we don't like the state of mind we're in, we can choose another. All that's required is to sit quietly and take a few deep breaths. As we calm ourselves and move our attention to that place where we are at peace; we make contact with the wise being who lives inside us and is always serene. Then we realize we have freedom of choice. We can choose from a wide range of emotions. We can choose how we want to respond to the events around us; we can connect to the wisdom of the universe.

The more we practice going inside to contact our inner guide, the easier it will be to remember we have a choice.

There is a place inside me that is always calm, peace-
ful, and serene. It is my center. It is the home of my
inner guide. I go there many times a day.

Children tend to die with greater softness and ease than adults. Perhaps because they are not so involved themselves with attempting to control the universe, there is not so much tension in their minds.
— *Stephen Levine*

Even in their dying, children have something to teach us — how to live with greater softness and ease.

Our culture puts a premium on control. Our heroes are the businesspeople who know what they want and know how to get it. They're always in control. They're also a myth. Nevertheless, many of us beat ourselves up trying to become that in control "hero."

Surrender, the alternative to control, doesn't get much cultural support. Yet, when we surrender, we gain incredible strength — not tense strength, but subtle, flexible strength, like the ocean. We step into the world of real heroes when we surrender, we align our will with a higher purpose. When we stop trying to control the world, we live with greater softness and ease.

I let go of worry and control. I willingly surrender to the flow of the universe. Right action happens easily and effortlessly.

*Death is not the enemy; living in constant
fear of it is.*

— *Norman Cousins*

An irony about AIDS is that if we want to go on living, we need to think about our dying. It would seem like the last thing we would want to do; it would seem like we would want to keep all thoughts of death away from us. But until we make peace with our dying, we aren't free to go on living.

The point is not to accept that we will die from this disease. The point is to accept that we could die from this, or a lot of other things, and to bring up our feelings about that.

Fear of death is the ultimate shadow, but it is only a shadow. Like all shadows, fear of death disappears when we shine the light of our attention on it. We may be able to do this on our own, or we may want some help. However we do it, the wonderful result is that when we lose our fear of dying, living is more fun.

Today I will face any remaining fear of death that I may have and I will let it go. When I am not afraid to die, I am free to live fearlessly.

Clap your hands, all peoples!
Shout to God with loud songs of joy!
— Psalms 47:1

Making noise is great therapy. Opening our mouths and letting out sound starts movement. A vibration begins and all the things we want to let go of can start to move away from us — all the anger, hurt, and resentment.

All of us have unexpressed feelings stuck in our bones, tissues, and muscles, and they need to be released. They block expression and creativity, and make us sick.

Singing, dancing, and shouting helps release those old feelings. Inside all of us are songs, dances, and shouts wanting release. The more of them we let out, the better we feel. Whenever we have an opportunity to dance, sing, and shout, we ought to take it.

Even if we get lots of support for being quiet and complacent good boys and girls, that's not always the best way to heal. It's often better to make noise, shout out loud, dance, and shake. The more we release, the better we feel.

Today I will ask the holy spirit in me to start my body moving and vibrating and shaking and dancing and letting go of everything that blocks my healing.

The bottom line for everyone is, "I'm not good enough."

— *Louise Hay*

The belief that we are not good enough is the basic bad attitude that causes us pain, guilt, shame, and fear. It weakens our body and makes us vulnerable to disease.

Luckily, it's only a belief — something we have the power to change. We start changing it by being honest about what we believe. If we believe we aren't good enough, we own up. Then, we let the feelings that surround our beliefs surface. How do we feel when we say, "I'm not good enough"? What images come to mind? Why aren't we good enough?

Finally, we admit that we were wrong about ourselves. The truth is, we are good enough, just the way we are. Period. Good enough for everything.

The antidote to all those years of poisonous shame is simple: We tell ourselves how beautiful, good, acceptable, wonderful we are right now. As often as we can, we take Louise Hay's advice, we look at ourselves in the mirror and say, "I love you."

I love and accept myself just the way I am. I open to receive all the blessings of the universe. All that is mine by divine right now comes to me in totally harmonious ways.

I knew I was gay from the time I was eight years old. I never felt very comfortable with that fact because of my Catholic upbringing. I felt I had no self-worth and no chance for a happy life.
— *Mark Christopherson, person with AIDS*

Many of us made up our minds when we were children. We decided against ourselves; we believed we had to settle for less than happiness. Unfortunately, many of those judgments now keep us from blossoming into all that we can be.

Some of us judged that we could never be well, really healthy. Or we judged that we could never have satisfying relationships. Or that we'd never get our needs met. It's time to decide again. It's time to judge for ourselves in every area of our lives.

Nothing is more important to our healing than reversing those old judgments. We need to communicate our new belief to every cell in our body: we can be happy; all our needs can be met. Every part of us needs to radiate with our newfound self-esteem and hope.

The past no longer controls my beliefs. Old judgments slip away. I now know that, because of who I am, I can be happy in this lifetime.

*You must come to see every human being
including yourself as an incarnation in a
body or personality going through a certain
life experience which is functional.*
— Ram Dass

When we trust that a Power greater than ourselves
is guiding the universe, we are able to stop rebelling
against life. We operate out of a peaceful center.

When we look out at the world from this peaceful center, we become aware that we are more than
our bodies. We are beautiful beings of light, learning lessons, growing, and changing. We know that
our experiences, even the painful ones, have a
purpose and bring us to where we are now. We
know that AIDS serves a purpose too.

From that peaceful center, we become more aware
that God lives in us. We realize that accepting
our humanness helps us grow more divine. And
accepting the God in us helps us be more human.

*Help me view myself and the problems I face from my
peaceful center. Help me remember that I am a human
manifestation of a divine being.*

. . . as long as we identify with our ego or body/personality-self and believe we are limited by what we perceive in the physical world, we cannot experience our true reality — our spiritual self.
                              — Gerald Jampolsky

We are more than our bodies. We are more than flesh with little flickers of spirit inside. We are vast beings that exist beyond, before, and after our physical bodies.

The problem is, it's so easy to forget our spiritual, timeless selves. And once we forget, we take ourselves very seriously and worry that our needs won't be met.

When we forget who we are, we also forget other people are also spiritual beings. We end up feeling lonely, afraid, lost, and far from home. For many of us, AIDS is the crisis that helps wake us up and remember. As we remember our spiritual nature, we feel less afraid, less lonely, and our path home becomes more clear.

I am on a path home to remembering who I am. Every day more cells wake up and vibrate with new energy and new aliveness.

The first step toward change is acceptance. Once you accept yourself, you open the door to change. That's all you have to do. Change is not something you do, it's something you allow.
— *Will Garcia, person recovering from AIDS*

When we really want to change, we become willing to accept the truth. Like, I drink too much, or I'm lonely, or I'm afraid of dying. Denying the truth puts our feelings in a freezer and keeps us stuck.

Another way to stay frozen is to set conditions on our self-acceptance: "I'll love myself when. . ."

We need to give ourselves a cosmic break. Only then do we stand a chance. When we warm ourselves with loving self-acceptance for who we are right now — no ifs, ands, or buts — our problems start to melt.

Positive change is the natural result of love. All we have to do is allow love to flow through us. Acceptance is the key.

Today I will accept myself just the way I am. I will send loving acceptance to all parts of me, including the parts I want to change.

The overemphasis on bacteria has given rise to the view that disease is the consequence of an attack from the outside, rather than of a breakdown within the organism.
— Fritjof Capra

If, as a society, we spend all our time fighting "the virus," the so called cause of AIDS, we avoid the reason why our bodies break down and become susceptible to disease in the first place.

If, as individuals, we fall into the same denial trap, and run off in a desperate search for a cure, a pill, a wonder drug, we deny the lessons AIDS can teach us.

Disease susceptibility isn't only a matter of weakness in our bodies. It also involves belief systems, thought patterns, behaviors, and habits. It involves the activity of our minds and the awareness of our spirit.

We have control over whether we put all our energy into the search for a magic pill or whether we try to heal our whole self — body, mind, and spirit.

I will examine my judgments and beliefs, not just my blood. I will examine my feelings and my life history. I will allow my entire self, in all its many aspects, to stand in the light and be healed.

. . . recovery from codependency is exciting. It is liberating. It lets us be who we are. It lets other people be who they are.
— *Melody Beattie*

It's too painful to always be anxious because someone else, usually someone we love, isn't the kind of person we want him or her to be. When our serenity is dependent on someone else's behavior, we're in trouble.

If we're full of anxiety because other people aren't acting the way we want them to act, we've got a problem. If we wonder why people can't be more like us, we need to think again.

We deserve the freedom to be exactly who we are and other people deserve to be exactly who they are.

When we let go of our anger and resentment, and stop trying to make our feelings someone else's fault, we can start talking honestly about how we feel. We can focus again on *our* lives. When we stop trying to change other people, we can start making our lives exactly what we want them to be.

God grant me the serenity to live and let live. Help me recover my own life out of the chaos of unhealthy relationships and confusing feelings.

This year has been about recovery from AIDS fear. A year ago I hated to see the AIDS acronym in the paper. My eyes would swim and I would look away because I was sure I had it and would die.
— David Grundy

For gay men, AIDS is our shadow. It follows us, lurks behind headlines, hounds us over the telephone, and jumps out at us from the television.

We've been haunted by AIDS for many years. But AIDS fear is not limited to the gay community, it's everywhere. And like all fears, AIDS loses its power when we face it and say, "Okay, show me what you've got."

Of course, what AIDS has is our fear of death. When we confront the possibility of our dying, AIDS loses its power. When we stop running, AIDS becomes a disease, a political issue, a challenge, something we can handle.

AIDS still may be our shadow, but it's a shadow we can live with, part of us that we can embrace, accept, and listen to for the lessons it teaches.

I can confront my fear by admitting, accepting, and loving that part of me that is afraid. I can confront my fear of AIDS by facing my fear of death.

We must appeal to other physicians to stop the gloom and doom stuff.
— *Nathaniel Pier, M.D.*

Amen. Stop the doom and gloom stuff. Right now. Of course, we have little control over what the great body of medical people say or do to others. We do have control over what they say and do to us. We can insist that there be no negative, hopeless prognosis based on the statistics around us. We can let them know that all death messages and beliefs that AIDS is always fatal are unwelcome and will be rejected. If they persist, we will part company.

AIDS is a fightable disease, treatable and manageable. That doesn't mean we'll live forever. It means we have an opportunity to heal and the right to try.

As we stand up for ourselves against negative beliefs, we allow power to run through us. When we refuse to submit to someone else's thinking, we stop being a victim and become powerful people.

I am an empowered person. I will not allow any doom and gloom AIDS hysteria in my presence. I believe that AIDS is fightable and treatable.

*First and foremost, leave your mind open
to possibility.*
— *George Melton, person recovering
from AIDS*

When our mind is closed to new possibilities,
opportunity could be furiously pounding on our
door but we wouldn't hear a thing. When our mind
is closed, we are blind to creative solutions, even
if they are as brilliant as ice castles in the sun.

But when we open our mind, we can hear soft
whispers and see faint images of hope. When our
mind is open, the slightest possibility can grow and
become living reality. When our mind is open, our
heart opens easily too. Our open heart can then
lead our mind into new believing, into wonderfully
new possibilities.

Every time we take a risk, or open up to others,
or go to a new support group, or learn about alter-
nate treatments, or hear what works for other people
with AIDS, our open heart leads our open mind
and we are living in love.

*My mind and my heart are open to the wildest possi-
bilities and the grandest opportunities.*

Numbers, science, and medicine all fail to answer a deceptively simple question: Why me?
— Tom O'Connor, person with ARC

Asking "why me?" can start us on a self-pity binge. We can stay in our anger, or resentment, or self-pity for as long as we think we need to. When we're ready to move on, the question remains: why me?

We may try to answer it by blaming ourselves and feeling guilty for our past behavior. Still the question remains. Once we forgive ourselves we discover that hiding behind our anger and guilt is our sadness and our grief, the pain we've been running from for so many years.

Finally, we realize that the running is worse than the pain and we surrender. We begin to cry, to release the tears that we've blocked with our guilt, anger, and denial. We let the healing power of tears wash over us. We listen and begin to hear the answer to "why me?"

I bless my anger. It tells me I am alive. I bless my sadness. It reminds me that I am real. I bless my confusion. Out of it comes clarity. I bless my tears. They heal me.

Our normal waking consciousness, rational consciousness as we call it, is but one special type of consciousness, whilst all about it, parted from it by the filmiest of screens, there lie potential forms of consciousness entirely different.
— William James

Our rational consciousness, or being aware of the world around us on a limited, operational level, can hide from us other ways of being aware. It is not the only state of being available to us.

We are all familiar with other forms of consciousness. Dreaming is one, deep meditation is another. And so is that creative, intuitive space just before sleep and just after waking. Close contact with nature can also put us in a special place of peace.

Living in these other states of awareness can be very healing. Our busy mind is given a rest, we are relaxed, and we are able to communicate feelings of peace, security, and well-being to our body. And our body responds.

Allowing ourselves time to meditate, dream, connect to nature, and be creative unites us and helps us heal — body, mind, and spirit.

I cross the flimsy barriers of consciousness easily and effortlessly. I am relaxed and my body is healing.

Now my Angels wear no wings of gold
You wear no robes so bright
For You're the father, the mother,
the sisters, and the brothers
Who held me through the Hell day
*   and night.*
— David A. Bergin, person with AIDS

AIDS is about families — our mothers and fathers, our sisters and brothers, our uncles and aunts, our children. Some of them hold our hands while we're in the hospital, some don't. Some are overcome with fear. Some overcome their fear.

Some of us are afraid to talk to them. We're afraid to be honest about our feelings, our sexual preference, our health. Still, many of us are moving past our fear and being honest with our families about who we are and how we feel.

Our need for family goes beyond biology. Our friends, people with AIDS and AIDS-related conditions, people from our support groups, lovers, and former lovers — they're all part of our family. It's a family we've built by being honest about who we are, how we feel, and what we need.

Today I pray for the courage to be who I am, true to myself, in the presence of my family. I also pray for the courage to ask for what I need.

And since the human body tends to move in the direction of its expectations — plus or minus — it is important to know that attitudes of confidence and determination are no less a part of the treatment program than medical science and technology.
— *Norman Cousins*

When we expect a positive result, we turn our body to the light. Our whole self follows the lead of our expectation. Every day, we can take inventory and ask ourselves, "What are my expectations?" Once we know, we can make adjustments to make sure we're pointed in the direction we want to go.

We also need to remember to surround ourselves with people who expect positive results — people who bolster our confidence and support us in our determination and recovery.

And we can be that kind of person for other people too. When we believe in miracles, we can be very influential members of someone else's recovery team.

———————————

Miracles happen in my life every day. I look for them; I expect them. They are nature's way of winking at me.

The human body has a natural propensity toward health. Always toward health.
— *Will Garcia, person recovering from AIDS*

What is my destiny, my purpose? What am I supposed to do with my life? These are hard questions. Even if we believe our life's purpose is to do God's will, we still have to figure out what that is, what that means.

So we look for answers from other people. For those of us who are gay or lesbian, or otherwise not part of the mainstream, some of these people are prejudiced against us. According to them, we're supposed to get sick and die.

If, however, we listen to our body, we will get a more informed, reliable, and loving answer. When we cut a finger, our body heals it. Automatically, God, nature, the universe, wants us to be whole and complete. God's will is that we be well.

That's as true for gay people, IV drug users, people of color, and people who test positive to HIV as it is for everyone else.

I ignore doom and gloom sayers and listen to my body instead. I focus on my health. My natural state is vibrant wellness.

Gradually, though, the addict learns to accept responsibility without denying the worth of his self. In this learning, a separation is made between the actions one commits and one's soul.

— David Mura

Whether we're addicts or not, most of us have done things that we wanted to keep secret. We've harmed other people and ourselves. Then, we hid our secrets in our heart and locked the door. We justified, and rationalized. We built thick walls around us and lived in fear of being found out. Finally, we lost ourselves in the deception.

Recovery means finding ourselves behind our guilt, shame, and rationalizations. It starts with honesty, telling our secrets, calling things by their right names, and owning up to the harm we've done.

The miracle is that when we unlock our heart and tell our secrets, we uncover our soul. When we let the secrets out, we let the light in. We experience the blessing of forgiveness and learn that who we are is not what we did.

I open my heart and release all my secrets. Light pours in and illuminates my soul. I know that I am forgiven.

The Hindus or Vedantists say that the Atman, or immanent eternal Self, is one with Brahman. Christians might say, "The kingdom of God is within you." Buddhists sometimes say, "You are the Buddha."
— From *Chop Wood, Carry Water*

God is not "up there" somewhere. God is here with us. Truth lives inside us. God is here, present in our hearts. When we feel shame and guilt, we forget who we are. When we expect attack, we forget that we are all one, that God is present in other people too.

The more we practice seeing God, the Buddha, the Goddess, Brahman, Christ, the Great Spirit, in everyone we meet, the easier it is to love them. The more we affirm and look for the presence of a Higher Power within ourselves, the easier it is to love ourselves.

I am the Buddha. I am Atman. I am filled with Christ consciousness. I am a child of the universe. All that I need I already have. I am surrounded in love and peace. I am.

*Grief can have a quality of profound heal-
ing because we are forced to a depth of
feeling that is usually below the threshold
of awareness.*

— *Stephen Levine*

AIDS has taken its toll and many of us are numb.
We've got a lot of grieving to do, some major weep-
ing and wailing. We need to open up to where our
pain lives, where our loss is stored. We need to cry
alone, and we need to cry together.

Even as we celebrate our living, we need to mourn
our losses. AIDS opens a great sadness for us as
individuals and as a community. To discount our
sadness, or to ignore it, is to deny ourselves the
opportunity to heal.

Personal grief opens us to being more fully
human; we become aware of how deep and far our
feeling goes, of how big we are. Community grief
joins us together and makes us stronger. Through
our grief, we become more vulnerable, more inclu-
sive, more alive than ever before.

---

*God grant me the place and space and time to
grieve. Through my grief, teach me about myself,
about how much there is of me. Through our grief, bring
us together.*

I do not limit God by seeing limitation in myself. With God and myself all things are possible.

— *Florence Scovel Shinn*

It's easy to fall into the trap of believing that because we have AIDS, ARC, HIV antibodies, or because of any number of other reasons, our possibilities are limited. After all, there are lots of people out there who believe in only very limited possibilities for people with AIDS, just as there are people who believe there are only limited possibilities for people of color, women, or gay people. It does not need to be true.

Because we're connected to the limitless source of all power, our possibilities are unlimited. Miracles are the natural function of this higher power; together we are a team.

To free ourselves from limitation, we must remember our connection and surround ourselves with people who believe in us. The best way to find those people is to be that kind of person — hopeful, unlimited, expansive.

I am unlimited. I am joined to the source of all supply. All things are possible. All things are possible.

*By learning to contact, listen to, and act
on our intuition, we can directly connect
to the higher power of the universe and
allow it to become our guiding force.*
— Shakti Gawain

Of course, our ego will not like it. Ego wants to
be in control and won't be happy with a decision
to turn control over to a Higher Power.

But ego will get used to it. Besides, how helpful
has ego been lately anyway? Ego keeps us alone,
separate, afraid, and on the defensive. Ego tells us
that our character defects make us who we are; ego
warns that if we listen to intuition, we'll dissolve
into cosmic conformity or misty nothingness.

Ego is wrong. The more we contact our intuitive
knowing, the more genuine, honest and true to our
unique selves we actually become. Instead of being
isolated and alone, we feel connected, part of the
whole. We realize that "the higher power of the
universe" is not some distant, way-up-in-the-sky,
other-than-us force; Higher Power is personal and
present. Higher Power lives in us and speaks to us
through our heart. It is at once "mine" and at the
same time it is universal and shared by everyone.

*I sit still and listen to my inner voice. I am guided by
my intuition and act in harmony with the universe.*

*As your faith is strengthened you will find
that there is no longer the need to have
a sense of control, that things will flow as
they will, and that you will flow with them,
to your great delight and benefit.*
— Emmanuel

No doubt about it, AIDS causes a lot of uncertainty, stress, and worry. But so does the stock market. So do many things. No matter what we're worrying about, the issue is the same: we want control; we want things to go our way. And if they don't, we become afraid, stressed, and frustrated.

There is an alternative to worry and fear: acceptance and faith. We accept that we aren't in control; we don't know what's going to happen. We have faith that no matter what, we are protected and cared for by a Power greater than ourselves. So, we aren't afraid. Instead of trying to control everything, we surrender. We take a leap of faith.

I am finding, to my great delight and benefit, that going with the flow is easier than I thought and more fun than I imagined. Though life is uncertain, I know I am protected and cared for by a Power much greater than myself. That Power is directing the flow.

November

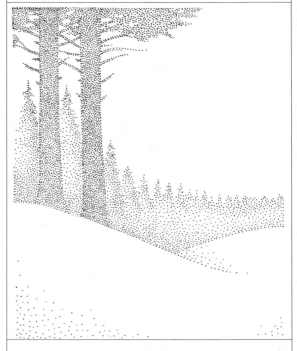

I honor the memories of those of us who are gone and I bless and honor the presence of those among us who stand like evergreens.

An innocent, inquiring, open mind is a
prerequisite for healthy living. If you are
open to new possibilities in your life, then
that alone will give you access to those
possibilities — readiness is all.
— *Deepak Chapra, M.D.*

If we decide ahead of time that doors are shut
for us, we'll probably find them shut. If, however,
we believe all things are possible, doors swing open
that we wouldn't even see otherwise.

We acquired most of our beliefs when we were
very young. Many of us, because we are gay, or
black, or female decided early on that lots of doors
were closed to us. All of us have felt shut out in
some way or other. When we did, we acquired
a belief.

Our task, now, is to uncover the negative beliefs
that keep doors shut for us and replace them with
the positive belief that new possibilities are always
open to us.

I open to all the wonder and bounty the universe has
to offer me. I am innocent and pure. I am a child of God.

"You mean that not caring about our brothers is one of the causes of sickness?"

"Exactly," answered the old man, *"not caring for one another has always caused sickness among a People. Caring is the only way to end sickness completely."*

— *Hyemeyohsts Storm*

There's a whole lot of caring going on among people with AIDS. All of us living with AIDS are part of a great move back to remembering who we are, to remembering that we are not alone, isolated or separate, to remembering that we are all one people.

However, there is a whole lot of caring that still needs to be done. There are still people with AIDS dying alone and living alone. There are children with AIDS abandoned to hospitals where they deteriorate because they aren't touched or held enough. There are gay people living in fear and homophobia and IV drug users living in the daily terror of addiction. There are mothers with AIDS who need love, acceptance and support. And there are mothers of people with AIDS who need support too.

Help me to care for all my brothers and sisters. Help me to remember we are the same person, one people. Bless us all.

Focus is important. Focus on those parts of yourself that are working. Look at yourself as someone whose body is in the process of healing. Concentrate on the positive parts.

— Will Garcia, person recovering from AIDS

Attention is like a big electrical cable. Energy and power flow through and along the path on which it is laid. The more we focus our attention on vital health, the more energy moves there.

Right now, all at once, in millions of places in our body, cells are regenerating. By placing our attention on those cells we give them an extra boost. We enliven ourselves and channel more healing energy.

That kind of focus works on our emotions too. Even when we feel filled with fear, we aren't. Some part of us is filled with love. When we focus our attention there, our love expands and our fear recedes.

How we see ourselves often depends on where we look, where we focus our attention.

Today I remember that I have power over my attitude. I focus on the positive and channel light through the magnifying glass of my attention. I am on fire, alive and aglow.

*You are used to listening to the buzz of
the world, but now is the time to develop
the inner ear that listens to the inner world.
It is time to have a foot in each world, and
it can be done.*

— *Bartholomew*

When we walk down a street or enter a strange
room, we automatically scope it out to find out how
safe it is, who's there, and what people are doing.
We gather information. We have trained ourselves
to listen and observe.

In the same way, we can train ourselves to learn
about the intuitive, nonrational, spiritual world. The
more we learn about this world, the more we come
to understand how important it is to our survival.

One way to turn our attention toward this world
is meditation. Whether we sit cross-legged, relax
by lying flat on the floor, take long walks, gaze at
candles, or listen to music, the point is to calm ourselves and change our channels from the outer
world to the inner world.

Through meditation we consciously improve
our contact with our spiritual self, our guide and
we discover that living in the material world is easier
when we're listening to both channels.

Help me to listen with my inner ear.

I realized I have choices. They're like a huge field of beautiful flowers and I get to pick the ones I want. It doesn't matter so much what I choose, as long as I make a choice.

— Stephen Fish, HIV positive

I can choose to smile or frown. I can choose to stay in fear or move in love. I can be positive or negative. I can choose my attitude.

And I can choose my dreams. I can choose all the elements that go into my picture of what I want my life to be — the people, the career, all of it.

I can choose my doctor, my treatment, my program for recovery. I can hang on to my fears and old habits or let them go. I can go it alone, or I can ask for help.

I can choose to wait and get sick, or I can take action and choose from among a huge number of immune-building alternatives.

And as long as I remember that I have choices, I know that I am neither a victim nor helpless.

Every day, and especially when the world looks gray and dull and I feel trapped and stuck, I will visualize a field of beautiful flowers and remember that I have choices.

God loves the world through us.
                    — *Mother Teresa*

One of the tenets of Alcoholics Anonymous is that you can't keep it unless you give it away. A.A. started when one alcoholic tried to help another alcoholic find a spiritual path out of drinking. In the process they both stayed sober.

What we give we get back. When we give love we receive love. When we give strength, we get strength because we are all connected, part of the same whole. When we give love we're loving ourselves.

We get into trouble when we become attached to the results of our giving. It means we've decided to run the show. Then our giving has strings attached that return as resentment, bitterness, and disappointment.

What a relief to let go of our attachments and realize we aren't responsible for any outcomes. All we have to do is be willing to allow love to flow through us.

I am a clear channel for love. Love moves through me and I am healed.

*Often I am scared and lonely, squeezing
love like a stingy old man with toothpaste.*
— *Tom Young, person with AIDS*

Love is infinite. We can't use it up, but we can
be blind to its presence. When we are scared and
lonely, it's hard to see or feel the healing love that
surrounds and protects us.

Fear pulls a film over our eyes, which keeps us
from seeing who we are. Fear would have us believe that we are merely a body. Fear says there is
no God, we are all alone, and there is not enough
love in the world to go around.

Fear is wrong. We are so much more than our
bodies and personalities. We are also spirit. And
each of us is capable of generating oceans of love.
All we have to do is recognize that we are plugged
into the source of unlimited love. And, because love
expands, the more we extend love, the more love
there is to share. So, we needn't be stingy. We can
use as much love as we possibly can today and still
be adding to the love that exists in the world.

---

*Today I imagine love in the form of a golden white light.
I am filled with this light and radiate it wherever I go.*

Aliveness is not necessarily about feeling better, curing ills, or solving problems; it is about feeling more, being in touch with a larger dimension of awareness.
— *Richard Moss*

Illnesses that confront us with the possibility of dying are especially good at raising our consciousness. Facing death causes us to become more open to experiencing a world that exists beyond what we can see and touch, a world of spirit and light.

Once we sense our connection to that world, we can steadily increase our awareness. All we have to do is ask and we will awaken to greater awareness of a world where we are always alive, always connected to everything and everyone.

Any illness, including AIDS, that helps us connect to our spiritual side can be thought of as a gift. Especially if we let go of all judgments about what successful healing is and all judgments about where we "should be" by now and trust that we are always exactly where we need to be.

I let go of all judgments about my healing and open to a "larger dimension of awareness."

*Look into your eyes and say out loud,
"I love you, I really love you." Do this first
thing in the morning and last thing at
night. Do it often during the day.*
— Louise Hay

Our words are powerful. What we say can be
harmful or healing. Unfortunately, most of us
are constantly criticizing ourselves. Our internal
dialogue goes something like, "You don't look right.
You need to gain weight. You don't meditate enough.
You aren't good enough."

Luckily, self-criticism is just a habit, and we can
change our habits. We can choose words of praise
instead. We can make a habit of speaking powerful
words of healing. We can choose immune-building
words that are more powerful than any drug. The
most powerful of them all are *I love you.* Saying those
powerful words, often and out loud, looking straight
into a mirror, can reverse past criticism.

I forgive you are three more healing words that
work best when looking into a mirror. Looking into
a mirror and saying positive things makes self-love
a practice and, soon, a habit.

---

*Today I will use a mirror and practice self-love. I will
look into my own eyes and say, I love you. I really, really
love you.*

*By attending meetings on a regular basis,
we can begin to sit with the painful feelings we have been running from.*
— Handout from an Adult Children
of Alcoholics meeting

When we sit still and listen to other people talk
about their lives, we begin to have feelings about
our own story. We look around and begin to realize that we are not alone and that it may be safe
now to feel.

And we discover that people don't die from their
feelings. So now, instead of running away, medicating
ourselves, or getting stuck in denial, we just sit still
and listen and feel. And somehow, we get the
courage to return again next week. And even when
we are overwhelmed, we at least know that these
are our feelings. Which must mean that we exist.
We are alive. After so many years of not feeling, this
is a miracle.

Miracles are the business of recovery and support groups. They happen because we meet with
others and become willing to experience our
feelings.

---

*God grant me the courage to get help. I am tired of
running from myself. I am tired of being afraid. Thank
you for providing the support I need.*

Detaching doesn't mean we don't care. It means we learn to love, care, and be involved without going crazy.
— *Melody Beattie*

It's easy to go crazy over AIDS. Our friends, lovers, and family members can be difficult and need a lot of attention. Their behavior can sometimes make us crazy.

Of course, they can't make us crazy. Only we can do that. When our feelings are determined by what other people say or do, something's wrong with us — not them.

When we find ourselves letting others decide how we feel and think, it's time to detach and let others be responsible for their lives. It's time to mind our own business, our own happiness.

Detaching doesn't mean we cut people out. It means we stay present and loving without thinking we have to fix or manage the people around us. It means we stop trying to save people from the consequences of their behavior. Best of all, when we detach, we stop taking ourselves so seriously and start having more fun.

Today I will let go and let God. I will remember my friends are connected to the same source of divine energy I am.

Yoga is the method by which the restless mind is calmed and the energy directed into constructive channels.
— B. K. S. Iyengar

When we practice meditating, the practice becomes the thing itself. Doing it is the benefit. We meditate in order to meditate, not to train for some spiritual competition. If, for a moment, we are able to calm our restless mind and still our body, we are at our goal; we are meditating. Even if we can't seem to still ourselves, we are at our goal, meditating.

We need to give ourselves credit for our accomplishments. We can be so focused on striving and becoming that we miss the arrival. We cannot do better than be present in this moment. If we are here now, we are here now. That is everything.

However we choose to meditate, whatever form we use, all we have to do is practice. Practice without judgment, practice without attachment, practice with acceptance.

Today I will practice what I do to calm my restless mind. I will practice and that will be enough.

> *Yesterday is but a dream, tomorrow is but*
> *a vision. But today well lived makes every*
> *yesterday a dream of happiness and every*
> *tomorrow a vision of hope. Look well,*
> *therefore, to this day.*
> — *Sanskrit proverb*

Those of us recovering from addiction know the value of living one day at a time. And all of us, regardless of whether we are recovering from addictions, know how scary the future sometimes looks. We wonder if we're up to it, if we've got what it takes to make it through so much uncertainty. Living one day at a time can break the uncertainty into manageable pieces.

One day at a time living is a good answer to AIDS too. Actually, it's a good answer to life. The past is gone for all of us, and none of us know what tomorrow will bring. We have today. When we focus on living well today, we can do better than just get through the day; we can have full, rich days.

If we want to make this day really special, we can ask the little child inside us what he or she wants. We can treat today like an important occasion. Because it is.

I won't worry about yesterday or tomorrow. I will do at least one thing my inner child wants to do today.

Medical schools not only generate stress but neglect to teach their students how to deal with it.

— *Fritjof Capra*

Reducing the unhealthy stress in our lives is important to all of us living with AIDS. Our immune systems shut down when we're overly angry, afraid, or agitated. Our body works best when we are calm.

So we're learning about meditation, support groups, phone therapy, prayer, and Twelve Step groups. We're learning to let go of old anger and resentment. We're saving our lives.

We're not only students; we're also teachers. We're teaching our doctors to cure by using stress reduction techniques.

The AIDS drama is filled with heartbreaking stories, and our doctors are involved in most of them. Too often, they work too long and too hard without ever getting an emotional break. We can help by acknowledging our doctor's humanity every time we see him or her. We can treat our doctors as equals instead of father figures or gods.

Most of all, we can keep reducing stress and anxiety in our lives. Serenity is contagious.

Today I pray for peace of mind for all AIDS doctors.

God is our refuge and strength, a very present help in trouble. Therefore we will not fear.

— *Psalms 46:1-2*

Channeled through our heart, divine help is always available. But if we stay in our heads, intellectual and logical, help has a hard time reaching us.

Our heart already knows God. If we allow ourselves, our hearts can lead us to an understanding that our head is happy with too. An understanding that is good and right for us — God as we understand God. For many of us, it takes a crisis to bypass our head and go straight to our heart for help. We needn't feel any shame about waiting until we're in trouble. God doesn't mind. That's what crises are for.

As we are comforted in our difficult times, we learn to trust in the constant presence of a Power greater than ourselves. We learn that we don't have to wait until times are bad to ask for refuge and strength. Every day, we can surrender our lives to that care and protection.

The light of God surrounds me. The love of God enfolds me. The power of God protects me. The presence of God watches over me. Where I am, there God is.

There is not a heart that exists...
that, if it were assured of safety,
would not open instantly.
It is all an issue of fear.

— *Emmanuel*

So many of us keep the truth of our lives locked in our heart because we decided it wasn't safe to be honest.

We may know exactly when that happened and have clear memories of physical or sexual abuse, neglect, or poverty. More likely, our memories are foggy and we can't remember. We can, however, reconnect with the feelings we experienced way back then, feelings that caused us to judge the world as too hostile and unsafe for us.

And so we put on our armor. The armor protected us for a while, but now it is too heavy. So we start to tell our story. We let out our secrets. We take off our armor and learn that when we are honest about who we are, we are strong and safe.

My defenselessness is my strength. My honesty is my freedom. My heart is open to the light.

And I walk a pathway of angels
Who are sent to comfort me
And each step I take
And each hand I take
I am touched
I am healed
And set free.
  — David A. Bergin, person with AIDS

We determine the quality of our life. The kind of day we have is determined by our point of view. For example, rather than seeing those around us as threatening or harmful, we can imagine they are angels sent to guide us and help us on our way.

As we come to believe that one way God works is through the people in our lives, it becomes easier to see people beyond their shortcomings. When we recognize them as they really are, their touch does heal. When we let these angels take our hand, we are open to receiving all the love of God's universe. We complete a circle of love that heals our heart and sets us free. Best of all, we become grateful. Gratitude is a gift we give ourselves when we choose to see others as they really are.

Help me see the spirit essence, the angel character, of all the people in my life. Help me reach out for their healing touch.

A perfectionist never has developed an internal sense of how much is good enough.
— *Gershen Kaufman*

Many of us who grew up in dysfunctional families never learned when to say, "stop," "no," or "that's enough." We never knew what was enough fun or enough pain. We were never sure when our achievements were good enough.

Now, as adults, we have a hard time knowing what's enough. In relationships, we wonder if we're paying enough attention to the other person or if our partner is paying enough attention to us. At work, we're never sure if what we do is good enough. Our perfectionism keeps us from enjoying our lives. We still think our value depends on what we do. And we can never be, do, or have enough.

What we didn't learn as children we now must teach ourselves — our worth isn't dependent on our achievements. We are totally acceptable the way we are. We can relax. We are already perfect examples of complete, whole human beings. We are enough.

When I am anxious because I fear I must do better or more, I will calm down and know that I am complete, whole, and always enough just the way I am.

Seen in its true light, everything is a test. And so, focused in the present, sincere towards others and trusting in your process, know that you cannot fail.
— Ralph Blum

Life is full of tests; tests about money, relationships, sex, sickness... Often these tests aren't as paralyzing as the fear that accompanies them. When we're afraid we think of ourselves as a particular body or personality. We feel vulnerable and fear judgment and failure.

But this is our life. How could we possibly fail life? Even death is not a failure. It is only another transition, another opportunity to learn and grow.

As we remember that we are not just our bodies but also mind and spirit, we throw out all ideas of failure, guilt, blame, and judgment. We remember that all we have to do is live, as best we can, one day at a time; we're only responsible for our effort. Our Higher Power, the Spirit of the Universe, will take care of the outcomes, so we cannot possibly fail.

I love and accept the process that I call my life. I am on a grand adventure.

One thing the AIDS crisis has done is allowed a lot of people to start doing what they really want to do.

— Gary

AIDS has transformed many of us, motivating us to do now what we've always wanted to do. We're finding jobs we like, starting projects we're committed to, traveling, and taking risks.

This isn't always easy. It means knowing what we want from life. It also means we need to check in each day with ourselves to ask, "Is this right for me? Am I now being true to myself? What do I really want to do today?"

Although we may have doubts, if we are being true to ourselves, signs will appear to show us that we're on the right path. Doors will open that we didn't know were there.

We may make a few mistakes, get on the wrong train, try the wrong path. But none of it will be wasted. Everything we do will be a part of being true to ourselves. We need not be afraid.

I trust my higher self to support me in being true to myself. Doors open for me, and I happily walk through them. My life is an exciting adventure, and I am pleased.

They were still close enough to having been born to remember in their deep dreams the perfect stillness of all things. They did not doubt that, by believing, they could rise and travel through the air, leaving at their feet a blurring trail of light like a long white gown.

— *Mark Helprin*

Little children know they can fly. They don't doubt their imaginations and magical abilities. Little children are believers.

We were believers too. But as we got older, we stopped believing, our imaginations got dull. Our healing involves recovering our ability to believe. We need to believe that we have the power inside ourselves to heal and to recover from any disease, including AIDS.

Through our restored imagination, through the power of believing, and through our collective energy and love, we are learning to rise and travel through the air. We are confronting the general agreement that AIDS is hopeless and we are changing it. We are making AIDS fightable, treatable.

I am regaining my natural ability to imagine and believe. I let doubt disappear into nothingness. I am a believer.

. . .for in every adult there lurks a child — an eternal child, something that is always becoming, is never completed, calls for unceasing care, attention, and education. That is the part of the human personality that wants to develop and become whole.

— *Carl Jung*

If we don't pay attention to our inner child, he or she will act out the issue we're avoiding. In other words, we end up with some crisis that finally gets our attention. Sometimes it takes a big crisis like AIDS to get our attention because we're afraid to face our neglected inner self, that part of us that is innocent, loving, and beautiful. The good news is this: when we do start paying attention, we learn that we are not dead inside. We survived.

While we can't make up for all those years of neglect, starting now we can be kind, thoughtful, patient, protective, wise, and gentle parents to the little child inside.

Today I will be a wise and loving parent to the child who lives in me.

As far as the laws of mathematics refer to reality, they are not certain; as far as they are certain, they do not refer to reality.
— *Albert Einstein*

Science gives us symbols for reality. That's all. Physics, biology, mathematics, medicine provide only approximations of how our world is perceived. We sometimes forget this, especially when it comes to AIDS.

We could update Einstein's idea and say that as far as medicine refers to AIDS, it is not certain. As far as it is certain, it does not refer to AIDS. The truth is, modern medicine does not have a corner on understanding how the human body works.

Science can help us, but healing happens inside our bodies, not in a test tube. The more we pay attention to our bodies and the more we listen to our intuition, the closer we come to understanding our reality.

I am grateful for medicine and science and listen to what they have to say. I also take counsel with my self, my body, my intuitive knowing, and my Higher Power.

Stop being obsessed with perfection and orderliness and leave room for flexibility in your life. Be spontaneous again....
Play more at the game of life.
— Susan Smith Jones, Ph.D

Because of the uncertainty of AIDS, we sometimes try to make our lives as neat and tidy and controlled as we can. Too often, we forget to have fun. We take ourselves too seriously, and we don't take time to play. We forget that playing is even an option.

That's when watching children play can help us. Children can teach us how to be spontaneous, how to do something that's not part of a plan. When children play, they are there in the moment fully enjoying what they are doing.

Being spontaneous means being present in the moment. It means accepting the chaos of life and not being afraid of it. It means knowing that behind the chaos is an orderliness that we aren't in charge of and we can't control. It means letting go and living now. Free.

Because the world is already perfect and orderly, I get to play in the flowing, streaming chaos of life. I live in the moment, always ready to try new things. I see a freshly born world every minute of the day.

Friends, lovers, family and/or support groups of other persons with AIDS are, in my opinion, crucial to any survival strategy. No one should go this hard road alone. Don't isolate yourself. Make contact with others.

— *Michael Callen, person with AIDS*

All of us living with AIDS need support. We need to avoid the trap of isolation. Fear sets that trap by telling us we'll be rejected if we ask for help, or by leading us to believe that we don't belong and don't deserve help. Besides, if we don't tell anyone how we feel, we don't have to admit our pain to ourselves.

We need to break the habits that fear uses to keep us isolated. We deserve to be listened to and understood. We deserve support in our pain and encouragement in our healing.

When we reach out to receive help, we discover that we also have lots of love to give. Just by opening up and sharing our feelings, we give someone else the courage to ask for help too.

When I admit that I can't do this alone, I gain incredible strength. God grants me the courage to reach out and ask for help.

Enthusiasm is one of the most powerful engines of success. When you do a thing, do it with all your might. Put your whole soul into it. Stamp it with your personality. Be active, be energetic, be enthusiastic and faithful, and you will accomplish your objective.

— *Ralph Waldo Emerson*

Most of us have never had a bigger challenge than AIDS. Suddenly, we're confronting this life-threatening disease that says, "Act now." And we think, yes, it could be a big mistake to procrastinate on this one.

So we go for it. We decide what we want and what kind of healing we need. We commit. Whether our goal is restored health, restored relationships, or both, we do it. Whatever our program includes — eating right, exercising, meditating, or spiritual study — we do it with all our might.

As we learn to live with AIDS, we learn to live in the present. We stop procrastinating about our lives. We learn that it's not just AIDS that's happening now. Life is happening now. And we can commit to life 100 percent.

I am energetic, active, and an enthusiastic believer. I am meeting the challenges of life, and I am exhilarated.

*. . . abuse is an act where power is used
to steal from another what can only be
given freely.*

— David Mura

We have a right to a true history of ourselves, a history that fully acknowledges any harm done to us. Because if we were physically, emotionally, or sexually abused, and deny the harm done to us, we discount ourselves. We continue a childhood message that says we aren't worth much.

What a mistake. We are each priceless beyond words. That's why we need to look at our past and try to tell our story, honestly, including the hurt, the sadness, the fear, the loneliness, and the rage.

If we can't remember very much, we can listen to other people's stories. When we identify with their pain, we can know that the feelings we are experiencing are true. We can trust our heart.

As we tell the truth, our secrets, we become free. We say, "No, it was not okay. Yes, it was a big deal. Yes, I'm sad and rageful too. Most of all, I'm relieved to finally be telling a true history of my life."

God grant me the courage to remember and the willingness to look back through the lens of my heart at the suffering of my childhood. Give me an honest history, so I can claim my soul.

And when the stars decide to roll you,
You won't be able to stop them.
Not with all the sadness in the world.
     — *Tom Young, person with AIDS*

Look at how our lives have changed just because of AIDS. Which one of us could have predicted the changes that have happened in each of us and in our community? So many deaths. So many tears. So much growth and maturity. So much forgiveness and reconciliation. So much healing.

Above all, we have experienced love more deeply than we ever believed we could. We have learned to accept love as well as give it. The stars really rolled us a good one, and here we are, being intimate, vulnerable, empowered, weak, strong, sad, mad, hopeless, and hopeful.

And nothing we do stops it. Right and left, we are given opportunities to learn and grow and create. No matter how hard we try to slow the process the stars keep pushing us, the energy keeps coming. We might as well let go and enjoy the ride.

I am pushed along and led forward. I am offered the grandest possibilities for growth and change, for being who I really am.

*. . . the underlying source of our basic guilt
is always the belief that we have "sinned,"
and the fear that God will attack and
punish us for our unworthiness.*
— *Gerald Jampolsky*

God does not punish or attack. God does not see
us as sinful. We see ourselves that way. Sometime
long ago, we may have fallen victim to the idea that
we were bad, unworthy sinners and deserved
punishment and death.

Whether we believe in God or not, that core belief
in guilt keeps us locked in fear. We feel dirty, and
nothing we do can make us clean.

Starting today, we can examine our thoughts and
actions and ask, "Does this bring me closer to
living in the light? Is fear present? Do I feel guilty?"

It's important to examine how we feel about AIDS
in that light. AIDS is not punishment, for we are
not guilty of any wrongs against God. We are
innocent, pure beings of light.

---

*I forgive myself for forgetting who I am and for wrongly
believing that I am guilty. I let go of the past and walk
in the light of God's unconditional love.*

That which is the finest essence — this whole world has that as its soul. That is Reality. That is Atman. That art thou.
— *Upanishads*

I am the soul of the world. I am that which is the finest essence. These are words we need to hear again and again. Knowing who and what we are restores us to sanity and harmony with all things seen and unseen.

Not knowing who we are, losing ourselves in the illusion of shame and fear, is insanity. Believing that we are unworthy is insanity. Seeing only a world of division, where we are separate and alone, is illusion and insanity.

We have spent enough time lost in illusion. We needn't wander there any longer. All we need to do is ask to be restored to sanity. All we need to do is ask for a pathway out of the world of illusion. In the asking is the answer.

I am the soul of world. I am that which is the finest essence.

December

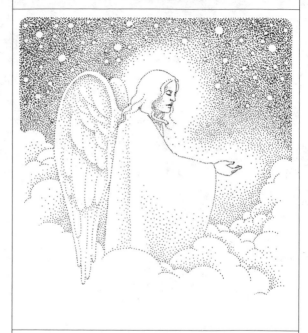

Help me see all the people I walk among as angels who are sent to comfort, guide and protect me. Help me reach out my hand for their healing touch.

*Bless the moment, trust yourself and expect
the best.*

— *Huna philosophy*

What good, simple advice. Yet many of us have
a hard time following simple advice. We're more
comfortable with complicated and confusing advice.

One reason is because we try to live in the past
or the future and we ignore the present. We predict
outcomes based on past events, old hurts, and fear.
When we live this way, the present is always suspect, ready to yield disaster. We can't trust anyone,
least of all ourselves. So we bounce back and forth
from the past to the future, worried and afraid.

When we keep things simple, we let the present
moment just be. We don't need to compare or
predict. We need only bless the moment and live
it fully.

When we keep it simple we trust ourselves. We
trust what's in our heart. When we keep it simple
we expect a good outcome without having to know
what it will be.

*I live in the moment, happy with myself and trusting
the universe to take care of me. My life is simple. My
heart is open.*

Walk in the sunlight every day for at least the few minutes it takes to remind your-self that the universe is our real timekeeper.
— *Deepak Chapra, M.D.*

We live in a world regulated by artificial sched-ules created for work and industry. By the time we're adults, a nervous timekeeper lives in our brains, keeping track of our deadlines and, if we let him, keeping us frantic most of the time.

When we give our timekeeper a few days off and step out of these artificial schedules, we have a chance to discover our personal rhythm. That's why after a relaxing vacation, we are peaceful and calm, we're in sync with ourselves.

We can live in that calm every day if we get out into the sunlight and pay attention to nature long enough to remember that we're connected to all things, long enough to realize that our deadlines are not to be taken too seriously, long enough to remember that there is a higher order at work, and according to that schedule, we're always on time and in the right place.

Today I remember that I am part of a bigger picture. Today I will keep my sense of humor about deadlines and demands. Today I will take the pressure off.

Once you begin to trust your heart
you will realize
that when something brings you joy and
fulfillment
it is the will of God
speaking through your heart.
— *Emmanuel*

Even when we decide to surrender our willfulness and go with the flow, we still have a problem. How do we recognize the flow? Put another way, how do we know what God's will is?

Some of us grew up thinking that doing God's will meant sacrifice and unpleasantness. We thought God was a stern father figure who scolded us when we had fun.

That was before we began to trust our hearts. Now, God as we understand God is a lot more fun. God's idea of a good time is often much better than ours.

In fact, the hardest part about doing God's will is letting go enough to have a good time. God, we have come to believe, wants us to be joyful and fulfilled. And we can find our way to that place of joy and happiness by letting our heart lead the way.

It's easy to pray, "Thy will be done," because I know that God wants me to be happy, joyous, and free.

*The press says that this is the one disease
in all the world you can't fight. I know how
brainwashed I am. I listened to them for
four to five years without defending myself.*
— Tom Young, person with AIDS

The good news is out. AIDS is a survivable disease. As treatments improve and we continue to
survive, more people realize that though still life-
threatening, AIDS is not always fatal.

We are moving toward a more hopeful attitude,
and we need to hear about it every day. We need
to listen to the voice of hope, hear about success,
and find out why people are surviving. We need
big doses of support to counteract all the bad news
we heard before we started to defend ourselves.

We need to stand as a grand, massed choir and
sing out our affirmations loudly. We need to give
ourselves permission to live and affirm that AIDS
is a treatable, fightable disease.

*I give myself permission to treat and fight this disease.
I give myself permission to win.*

Relinquishing control is the ultimate challenge for the spiritual warrior.
— *Ralph Blum*

We are by nature trusting, but from the moment we are born, we start to lose trust. Little by little, or in traumatic big jumps, our parents, brothers or sisters, teachers, adults, friends, let us down. So we decide the world isn't a safe place and people are not to be trusted.

We build defensive walls which keep control of our lives. And we survive. Until one day, we realize that we're no longer children and that our protective walls have become a prison and our controls don't work. The harder we try, the worse things get. Somehow, we have to learn to trust again. Somehow we have to let go of control. We have to ask for help.

Then, little by little feeling returns. Our tears and anger break down the walls of our prison and we step out into the sunlight. We let go of the controls, reclaim our innocence and trust again.

Today I pray for the courage to break out of the prison of isolation and let go of my controlling behavior. I trust that I am protected and cared for and know it is safe to walk in the light.

*I will not interfere with the working out
of another's difficulties, however dear
and close we may be to each other.
Detachment is essential to any healthy
relationship between people.*
— *One Day at a Time in Al-Anon*

Detachment sounds cold-blooded and uncaring
— until we begin to practice it. Then, we realize
that detachment allows us to be more loving to ourselves and others. When we detach from feeling
the need to control we make room for more love.

For those of us who too easily get enmeshed in
other people's lives, learning to detach can be very
affirming. It gives us the freedom to meet new
people without the fear of becoming overly or inappropriately involved in their lives.

When we detach, we learn to live and let live.
We're more able to listen because we don't feel
responsible for everyone's problems. We can help
without meddling.

We know that our problems have been our best
teachers and so we don't try to deny our friends
the opportunity to learn their lessons too.

*Every day I worry less about what's wrong with other
people and focus more on making my attitude loving,
hopeful, forgiving, and supportive.*

*If I participated in creating this experience,
I can participate in getting rid of it.*
  — *George Melton, person recovering
    from AIDS*

There seem to be two ways of looking at having
AIDS — through the eyes of a victim or with the
vision of someone who takes responsibility for his
or her life. Great power is available when we stop
being victims and start taking responsibility.

Unfortunately, in taking responsibility, we may
find ourselves saying, "It's my fault." To get out of
this dilemma, the first thing to do is dump all the
judging, blaming, and guilt. We're not bad people
for having AIDS.

Once we dump the judgment and guilt, we can
also let go of the victim attitude. Then, we begin
to feel the energy flow through us; we remember
we are connected to the source of all power. No
longer AIDS victims, we take control of our treatment and participate in our recovery.

---

*I trust myself to participate in my life. I am connected
to the source of all energy and healing power.*

There is no more certain poison for the self that internalizing rage and thereby fomenting bitterness with the self.
— *Gershen Kaufman*

The sound of a lion's roar is thrilling. He opens his mouth wide as the world and lets loose his rage, frustration, desire. We can all learn from Leo's example. We all have a buttoned down part of us that needs release. Most of all, we have rage caused by the indignities to our spirit that we suffer all through life: from the meanness of other children, to the disinterest and abuse of parents, to insensitive teachers, to the abuse of living in a noisy, polluted city. All this and more ought to have us roaring.

If we don't let it out, it turns bitter inside us. It can turn into depression or illness.

How do we get rid of it? Driving down the freeway with the windows rolled up screaming at the top of your lungs works. So does screaming into a pillow and pounding it with our fists. Whatever we do, we must roar. Roar on the street. Roar in our homes. Roar where we feel like it as long as we don't hurt anyone.

Today I will roar like an angry lion. I will let my rage out into the universe in ways that are totally harmonious for everyone concerned.

It's not just people with AIDS who need support; the family does too. I think I needed support more than my son.
— Linda, mother of a person with AIDS

We all need support. To get what we need, we may have to ask for it and seek it out.

We all need support from people who understand and care. That's why support groups and healing circles exist for everyone affected by AIDS: for families, for people with AIDS and ARC, or for people who test positive to the HIV virus.

Some of us may not find the support we need from traditional sources, which means we may have to look in new places and ask new people. But it's there if we look for it.

As we find the support we need and open ourselves to love and care, we learn that the distinction between patient and caregiver is artificial. We learn that the more we open to receiving love the more love we have to share — that giving and receiving are the same.

AIDS is teaching all of us how to care, how to ask for help, and how to accept loving support.

Help me accept my own human needs. Teach me to ask for help.

You are held in the hand of God and totally loved. And when that love can be received the circuit is complete.

— Emmanuel

Many of us experienced the grace of God in the miracle of gaining our sobriety. We had failed to stay sober until the grace of God entered our lives. It felt like being chosen, as if a beam of light shattered the darkness and enveloped us in golden white light.

But really, the light had never left us. It was just that our eyes were closed and we were blind to its presence. Until, one day, life became so bitter that we opened our hands and asked for help. The hand of God was always there; we just became humble enough to grasp it. Grace entered our lives when we became willing to accept it.

God's grace also works on all of the fear and loneliness surrounding AIDS. AIDS can serve a purpose: it can cause us to finally open our eyes to the light and extend our hand for help. All we are asked to do is complete the circle of love. Our job is to help God do God's job — extend love.

Today I open my hands and humbly accept God's love. I help keep the flow of love moving because I accept it for myself.

Being able to experience God as a loving force, and a light shining within me and throughout the universe at all times, is very different from my childhood concept of God as an old man with a beard, way up in the sky, distant and external, waiting to judge me.

— *Gerald Jampolsky*

There's no benefit in believing God is going to beat us up. If we still believe that, or any part of that, it's time to let those old ideas go.

Our judgmental gods are created by guilt. Guilt makes us believe that we are bad and deserve punishment, so we create a punishing god to punish us.

We have an alternative to guilt — love. Love tells us that we are innocent children of God, protected and cared for, deserving of all good things. Love teaches us that God is a force that lives in us and operates through us. God is present and internal.

Love asks us to open our hearts and accept our divinity. Through the eyes of love, we are able to see God in ourselves and everywhere we look.

I now release all ideas of a judging, punishing God. I gladly open my heart and joyfully accept the reality of my own godliness. God is light and love; so am I.

*AIDS is a disease caused by too little love
rather than too much sex.*
— Tom O'Connor, person with ARC

There's a lot of blame in the air that tries to make sex responsible for AIDS. The problem is, many of us are buying it. We feel guilty about the sex we had and the sex we have now. We wonder if we gave anyone AIDS.

Of course, we need to be careful and honest with our partners. But hanging on to this guilt is destructive.

Sex is a divine gift. Sex doesn't cause disease. Guilt, lack of love, anger, and hate can cause disease. They contribute to the stress that reduces the ability of our immune systems to resist disease and infections.

Guilt can also cause us to be abusive and mean to ourselves; we don't give our bodies the support they need to stay well and fight disease.

What we all need now more than ever is mental immunity against the invading armies of blame and guilt. We need to surround ourselves with white light, self-love, and positive affirmations.

I am grateful for being a sexual person. My sexual energy is pure and divine, highly charged, and healing.

I go to meet my good.
   — From a Unity Church pamphlet

Everywhere we go — into the next room, out the door, across town — we go to meet our good. We expect good results. We trust that the next moment holds good things for us.

The good we are about to receive belongs to us. We are simply accepting what is ours by virtue of being children of the universe, sons and daughters of the Mother/Father God. Every good thing belongs to us. We deserve every happy experience. All joy, light, and love are ours and part of us.

If that's true about leaving the house, it must also be true about dying. There, too, we go to meet our good. As we affirm our living each day, each moment, we can also affirm our dying. We can be ready to die with great expectation if we are ready to live that way too. Our dying and our living become the same — transitions from one now to the next now.

I will write it on my hand, put messages on my mirror, and signs on my door: I go to meet my good. I go to meet my good.

Done with awareness, life is letting go of
fears, letting go of guilt, letting go of limi-
tations, letting go of ideas that trap you
in the patterns of habit and do not leave
you free to be spontaneous in the moment.
— *Bartholomew*

We love to watch children and babies play because they are so right there in the moment. We
wish we could be like that — joyful, spontaneous,
present.

The good news is, we can. The first thing we need
to do is let go of the past. Fear is based on the past.
So is guilt. Habits are just the past repeating themselves in our bodies and minds.

The problem is, most of the time we are unaware
of our fear, guilt, or limiting beliefs. That's why
awareness is so powerful. When we bring our attention, our awareness to our negative thoughts, we
give ourselves the opportunity to say, "I let you go.
I no longer need you."

And when we bring our preoccupation with the
past to our inner self or Higher Power, fear and guilt
slip away. Old habits dissolve and disappear.

I am entirely ready to let go of all those things that
keep me from enjoying a true, spontaneous present.

Hospitals can be temples and dark moments doors to new potential, if only we will it to be so.

— *Richard Moss*

The most amazing transformations often happen when we feel most afraid and helpless. In those moments of darkness we experience the mystery of death and transformation. We die and are re-born. We crawl out of our brittle shell and enter the world again, pink and vulnerable. We discover our strength is in our defenselessness, not in the hard walls we put up to keep people away, not in our shell.

In the mystery of transformation, we experience forgiveness. All we need is to be ready and willing to let it happen. If we open to grace, it has a chance to enter.

Aware of this mystery, we know that we don't have to be face to face with death to be transformed. We don't have to wait for a crisis. We can ask for grace, healing, forgiveness, and love to enter our lives now. We can practice readiness always.

Doors of light now open to me and I know that I am forgiven. I accept the miracle of grace in my life and I am transformed.

Oh yes, I plan for the future. I plan to go to college. But I really just live one day at a time.
— *Ryan White, person with AIDS*

One thing AIDS can teach all of us is how to live one day at a time.

Remembering to live just today is a great help to those of us practiced at postponing our lives and our happiness. When we wait to live, we miss the chance to be here right now. When our lives are on hold, we get busy but we never get intimate because we can't be intimate in the future, only in the present. Only today.

Those of us recovering from alcoholism or addiction to other drugs learned to stay clean and sober one day at a time. Soon we learned that that's the best way to live anyway. Living with AIDS is like that too. All together it's too much. Broken into a day at a time, we can manage.

We still make plans — they keep us moving. But we live them and enjoy them one day at a time.

Today is a gift. Today I will let myself plan for the future and live in the moment. I only have to live this day. Nothing more is asked of me.

Being honest is the only way to enter the New Age.
— *Martenard, as channelled by Richard Wolinsky*

Honesty is a quality we are all born with but almost immediately begin to lose. We can best imagine what it was like to be totally honest by watching little children. They spontaneously express feelings of joy, anger, frustration, and sadness. When they want something they ask for it. If they don't want to do something, they say so.

We stopped being spontaneous and honest when we stopped feeling safe. Some of us got so lost in fear that we lost our ability to tell true from false. Many of us turned to alcohol, other drugs, and compulsive behavior — a world where honesty just got in the way.

When we start recovering from our addictions, we get reintroduced to honesty. We realize that the world doesn't cave in on us when we tell the truth. We slowly lose our fear of everyone and everything and begin to return to the sanity of little children who are able to express their feelings honestly.

I know that it is safe for me to be honest. I will be honest with myself, my close friends, other people, and my Higher Power.

Truly the light is sweet and a pleasant thing it is for the eyes to behold the sun.
— *Ecclesiastes*

The saints and sages, and the many people who have had near death experiences talk about being drawn toward the light. The light they describe is comforting, sweet, and pleasant, full of love and safety.

Somehow we believe this and know it to be true because the message we sometimes feel from people we love who have died seems to be, "Do not be afraid for yourself and do not grieve for me. I am very happy."

Still, there's no proof. And each time one of our friends dies, and we are confronted with death again, we wonder.

In quiet moments we can ask our friends who have passed over what we need to learn, what we need to know. The answer comes wrapped in gentleness, in a feeling of comfort, peace, and safety: We don't have to die to turn and face the light. We can turn our attention inward and ask the light to appear now. We can ask that our eyes be opened so that we can see the light that always surrounds us now.

In quiet meditation, like a flower in a field, I turn toward the light. The light is sweet, and I am safe and warm.

Children begin by loving their parents; as
they grow older they judge them; some-
times they forgive them.
— *Oscar Wilde*

To be free of the past and completely experience
the present, we need to heal all our relationships,
including those with our parents. Relationships that
still fester when we think of them keep us tied to
the past; they keep us from living in the present.

The key is forgiveness. The first step toward healing is to forgive ourselves for what we may have
done. The next step is to forgive our parents.
However, if we have never given ourselves permission to be angry with our parents, we may have
to be angry for a while. But we can move toward
forgiveness, even in our anger. If we can't forgive
now, we can be willing to forgive. We can want
to forgive.

As we forgive our parents, we claim complete
responsibility for our lives. We stop being victims
and begin to see how all the circumstances of our
lives have contained gifts and critical lessons,
especially the circumstances of our birth.

I want to forgive all the people in my life. I bless them
all and wish them well.

Because our representation of reality is so much easier to grasp than reality itself, we tend to confuse the two and to take our concepts and symbols for reality.
— *Fritjof Capra*

It's easy to forget that the diagrams of how our immune system works are only flat, one-dimensional attempts to represent something that happens on many dimensions all at the same time. It's also easy to turn Acquired Immune Deficiency Syndrome into HIV disease and then forget that it's something that happens to a whole person.

But we happen on many levels, many dimensions; we are not flat. We have depth and width and height and curves; we are whole. We are mind, emotions, and spirit, powerful forces that affect our physical body.

So if we want vibrant health, we must pay attention to our whole self and get everything moving. We must get beyond the initials to reality to our entire body, mind, and spirit.

I live in a many dimensioned world of reality. I allow my consciousness to include my whole, radiant, divinely human self.

I am Sure you have Seen a little Child or a Person who is Gentle, Stricken with Sickness and sometimes Crippled by it. This Happens more because of the People not Caring than because of the Haters.
— *Hyemeyohosts Storm*

We are all as gentle and innocent as children, but we have been hurt by uncaring behavior. We have been discounted and told we are not acceptable for being gay or lesbian, for being people of color, or for just being who we are. We have never felt the support of our People. Even more than open hatred, that neglect, that lack of caring causes sickness.

Caring means acceptance. Caring means supporting others as they are, not as we want them to be. Until we feel cared for, we never get a chance to be freely and spontaneously who we are.

Now the caring must begin. Now we must care deeply about ourselves, about the child inside us who needs to feel accepted and safe. We start by giving ourselves as much unconditional acceptance as we can. When we spread that to all those around us, everything we send out will return to us magnified. That is our task.

I am supported, accepted, and safe. The universe is a safe place for me to be exactly who I am.

His soul swooned slowly as he heard the
snow falling faintly through the universe
and faintly falling, like the descent of their
last end, upon all the living and the dead.
— *James Joyce*

Truth usually appears to us as a mystery unveiled for just a moment, showing herself only as a feeling of knowing. That feeling doesn't translate well into language. Sometimes great writers and enlightened sages can awaken a memory for us.

Truth appears when we grieve for friends and family who have died because of AIDS. We cry for ourselves and for them, for the living and the dead. Our tears are like the snow falling faintly in Joyce's beautiful story. Our tears do not seem to be caused by fear for ourselves, or regret, or pity for our friends. Our tears seem impartial and neutral as the snow. They just fall.

We cry because we feel some truth, and truth, like great art, makes us cry.

The truth is some of our friends are gone. They have passed over. They are experiencing the great mystery. And we are still here. And we don't know anything about dying at all.

Bless my healing tears of grief.

There is so much focus on physical thera-pies and yet much of the problem with AIDS is on spiritual and emotional levels.
— *Misha Cohen*

Am I spending all my time on my physical healing and neglecting my spiritual self? Am I neglecting my emotional self?

When was the last time I took a walk with a good friend and talked for a long time about myself? Am I aware of what I am feeling? Do I make phone calls, or do I wait for the phone to ring? Am I shut down emotionally? What do I feel right now?

When did I last pray? When did I last meditate? Have I been communicating with a Higher Power? Am I taking time to just be, just listen?

Whenever we take stock of ourselves, it's impor-tant to be honest. It's also important to be gentle and loving. This is not an opportunity to be mean and critical. It is an opportunity to make sure we're doing everything we can, emotionally and spiritually, to help us heal physically.

I give thanks that all my needs are being met — emotional, spiritual, and physical. I live in peaceful harmony — body, mind, and spirit.

Ultimately, it's a very loving act to trust people with your anger.
— *Twila Thompson*

Many of us don't express our anger because we're afraid it's going to hurt someone. We're afraid it will explode and the force of it will kill.

If we don't express it, the only place our anger can turn is inside. Unexpressed anger becomes repressed rage which can make us sick and depressed.

When we allow ourselves to be angry and express anger, it leaves and makes room for forgiveness and compassion. We stop hating ourselves for the emotions we feel, and we start trusting other people. We let ourselves be human beings with a full range of emotions. We let other people be human beings too, capable of surviving our anger, capable of loving us for who we are.

Anger released in the presence of love washes us clean of bitterness and hate.

I accept myself just the way I am, a human being who can get angry. I pray for help and guidance in expressing my anger in healthy ways that allow me to release it and move toward forgiveness.

*Heaven is the space within each one of you
that dances in the light.*
— Emmanuel

When we feel really connected, when something so special happens that we know we're on the right path, our feet start dancing all by themselves. Our whole body moves with joy.

Some songs do that. The music enters our bodies and we start to snap our fingers and dance. We know we're alive!

Because we have felt that vibration, we know it's possible to be spontaneously happy. And somehow we know that inside each of us is a place that's always happy, a place where we are always dancing in the light. And even if we feel lonely and far from home, we have a lifeline back to the source.

Heaven isn't out there in the future somewhere; it's now. When we choose to live in the present, each day is an opportunity to dance in the light.

Even when my faith is small and the light in my life is only a flicker, I will turn toward it and pray, "Please God, open a space for me to dance in the light."

When it is night
I put my hands together
Even when I'm far from belief
And my heart is dry and bound.
— Tom Young, person with AIDS

Prayer is most helpful when we're "far from belief." And we all know what it's like to be "far from belief," to be spiritually empty and feel so cut off that we despair. Those are the times that bring us to our knees, that force us to put our hands together in humility and honesty and ask for help.

We don't need great faith to pray. In fact, we don't need any faith or belief at all. We only need to point ourselves in that direction; we only need to be a little bit willing to believe.

That tiny bit of willingness that comes when we surrender ourselves in prayer is all we need to become aware of the love that surrounds and protects us. Slowly, we come to believe. Our eyes begin to open as if for the first time and we feel loved, protected, cared for.

As we move toward belief, we come to know that we have always walked in grace even though we were unaware of its presence.

Even when I am far from belief, I am not far from love.

People with AIDS...deserve to remain within our communal consciousness and to be embraced with unconditional love.
— The Bishops of the California Catholic Conference

We need to be vigilantly mindful that we are part of the whole community — all of us. No person or group of people is dispensable, or not included. Nobody is "them." It takes all of us to make a whole.

And though we need to speak out against fear groups who threaten us and want to isolate and quarantine us, we need to be even more mindful of our own self-hating thoughts. Our own racism, our own homophobia, our own sexism can be even more poisonous and harmful than the hate we receive from those who pander to fear. If we place ourselves outside the pale of human embrace, no one can reach us.

The best way to make sure we always place ourselves at the center of the whole, the best way to always feel loved, is to give love unconditionally. As we see others, so will we be seen.

As I give, so I receive. We all are one.

Come to the edge.
No, we will fall.
They came to the edge.
He pushed them, and they flew.
— *Guillaime Apollinaire*

It often takes a major crisis to bring us to the edge, that place where we are asked to take a leap of faith. Then, only when there seems to be no other choice, are we willing to close our eyes and jump.

Each time we jump, we find that when we give up control and choose to trust, we do better than merely avoid disaster; we discover we can fly. This is always the message of spirit: You can fly. You think you will fall. But when you surrender everything, you fly. You are so much more than you think you are.

Fear, however, tries to keep us away from the edge. Fear tells us the edge is dangerous. Fear imagines the rocks below. Fear believes we can't trust anyone or anything. Fear is mistaken. The edge is our friend and crisis is our beloved teacher, the one who pushes us off and teaches us to fly.

Grant me the courage to let go of my controls and fly. Help me remember who I am.

*A controller doesn't trust his/her ability
to live through the pain and chaos of life.
There is no life without pain, just as there
is no art without submitting to chaos.*
— Rita Mae Brown

What a relief to give up, surrender, let go. No more
having to be in charge all the time. When we stop
trying to control everything we take a giant spiritual
leap into freedom.

The truth is we can't control other people and
we can't control all the events in our lives. Sooner
or later, the realization dawns on us — we are not
in charge. So we might as well relax and start
enjoying the show.

When we surrender to the chaos, life becomes
a grand adventure instead of a frightening ordeal.
When we trust ourselves to survive what may come,
we are free to be spontaneous — funny, angry, sad,
sexy, loving, right, wrong.

When we trust enough to stop trying to control
the world, we loosen our grip, unhunch our shoulders, unclench our jaws, and open our hearts.

*I surrender all my problems and all my outcomes to
the care of a Higher Power. I am free to experience
the joy of living.*

You are worthy because you are.
— *Seth*

What a revolutionary idea. As children, most of us learned that we had to earn our worth through what we did, or how we behaved. So we tried to be good and accommodating. Or we figured what's the use and didn't try at all. Either way, we were acting out our belief that who we were wasn't good enough. We were what we did and we could never do enough, well enough, to be acceptable. Some of us dropped out, and some of us kept trying to be perfect.

Well, heck with those old ideas. We are worthy because we are. We deserve all good things because we are. We are totally, 100 percent acceptable, 100 percent of the time. Period. That's all there is to it.

To turn that idea into a deeply held belief, we may have to go back to our childhoods and give ourselves now whatever emotional support we didn't get then. If sadness from all those years of shame arises, we can welcome it and let the healing tears flow. That was then, this is now.

I am worthy because I am.

Where birds have been
Snow fills the nests again
Delicately white.

— *Gerald Vizenor*

The seasons remind us that everything changes. Everything comes into being and goes out of being. The circle turns.

The beginning of a new season is a good time to look back at our lives and notice changes. There are new people, new understandings. And people have gone, leaving only empty spaces to remind us they were here with us. The pain we felt has softened, but the hole remains.

There have been other losses too: ways of living that we put away, attitudes and beliefs that no longer fit us. We are different today than we were one year ago.

As we let go of a season, of a year, of a way of living, we turn and face the future again, renewed, confident, knowing we are in sync with nature — with the rhythm of change, transformation, death, and rebirth.

I am part of this ever-changing world. I let go of the old me. I live in the now with the new me. I live in harmony with the seasons and with the flow of life into new forms.

SUGGESTED READING

The following books have been helpful to me. I hope you find them useful too.

Bamforth, Nick. *AIDS and the Healer Within*. New York: Amethyst Books, 1988.

Bartholomew. *From the Heart of a Gentle Brother*. Taos, N.M.: High Mesa Press, 1987.

Bartholomew. *I Come as a Brother, A Remembrance of Illusions*. Taos, N.M.: High Mesa Press, 1985.

Blum, Ralph. *Book of Runes*. New York: St. Martin's Press, 1983.

DeRohan, Ceanne. *Right Use of Will, Healing and Evolving the Emotional Body*. Santa Fe, N.M.: Four Winds Publications, 1986.

Emmanuel's Book: A Manual for Living Comfortably in the Cosmos. Pat Rodegast and Judith Stanton, eds. New York: Bantam Books, 1985.

Gawain, Shakti. *Living in the Light*. San Rafael, Calif.: Whatever Publishing, Inc., 1986.

Hay, Louise L. *You Can Heal Your Life*. Santa Monica, Calif.: Hay House, 1984.

Jampolsky, Gerald G., et al. *Goodbye to Guilt: Releasing Fear Through Forgiveness*. New York: Bantam Books, 1985.

O'Connor, Tom. *Living With AIDS: Reaching Out*. San Francisco: Corwin Publishers, 1986.

Psychoimmunity and the Healing Process: A Holistic Approach to Immunity and AIDS. Jason Serinus, ed. Berkeley, Calif.: Celestial Arts, 1986.

Shinn, Florence Scovel. *The Game of Life and How to Play It.* Marina Del Rey, Calif.: DeVorss & Co., 1978.

Siegel, Bernie S. *Love. Medicine and Miracles.* San Francisco: Harper and Row, 1987.

Simonton, O. Carl, et al. *Getting Well Again.* New York: Bantam Books, 1984.

Spence, Christopher. *AIDS: Time to Reclaim Our Power.* London: Lifestory, 1986. (178 Lancaster Road, London, W11 1QU. Telephone: 01-221-6513.)

Surviving and Thriving With AIDS: Hints for the Newly Diagnosed. Michael Callen, ed. New York: People With AIDS Coalition, Inc., 1987. (Available through the National AIDS Network, 1012 14th Street, N.W. Washington, D.C. 20005. Free to people with AIDS.)

INDEX

Other titles that will interest you...

One More Day
Daily Meditations for the Chronically Ill
  by Sefra Kobrin Pitzele
  A book of meditations applying Twelve Step principles to the daily challenges presented by a chronic illness. *One More Day* can help us live well in the present, instead of focusing on the past or the future, whether we have personal experience with a Twelve Step program or not. These powerful meditations help us to accept our health-related limitations while encouraging us to adopt a program of living that emphasizes choice-making and a sense of personal independence. 400 pp. Order No. 5145

AIDS and Chemical Dependency
  by Dorothy Flynn
  All chemically dependent people need to know about Acquired Immune Deficiency Syndrome (AIDS). Without any hysteria or hype, this new pamphlet helps us replace fear with facts. It describes how to evaluate our risk for developing AIDS, and how to prevent getting and/or spreading it. Most importantly, this pamphlet describes how the principles of the A.A. program apply to life in the age of AIDS. 18 pp. Order No. 5211
